LEISURE PROGRAMMING
··· FOR ···
BABY BOOMERS

Lynda J. Cochran, PhD
Anne M. Rothschadl, PhD
Jodi L. Rudick, MAS

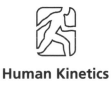

Human Kinetics

Library of Congress Cataloging-in-Publication Data

Cochran, Lynda J. (Lynda Jeanine)
  Leisure programming for baby boomers / Lynda J. Cochran, Anne M. Rothschadl, Jodi L. Rudick.
    p. cm.
  Includes bibliographical references and index.
  ISBN-13: 978-0-7360-7363-9 (soft cover)
  ISBN-10: 0-7360-7363-9 (soft cover)
  1. Recreation leadership. 2. Recreation--Management. 3. Leisure--Management. 4. Leisure--
Planning. 5. Baby boom generation. 6. Baby boom generation--Attitudes. I. Rothschadl, Anne
Marie, 1948- II. Rudick, Jodi L. III. Title.
  GV181.43.C63   2009
  790.06'9--dc22
                                        2008050149

ISBN-10: 0-7360-7363-9   e-ISBN-10: 0-7360-8745-1
ISBN-13: 978-0-7360-7363-9   e-ISBN-13: 978-0-7360-8745-2

The Web addresses cited in this text were current as of January 2009, unless otherwise noted.

Acquisitions Editor: Gayle Kassing, PhD; **Managing Editor:** Bethany J. Bentley; **Assistant Editor:** Anne Rumery; **Copyeditor:** Joyce Sexton; **Proofreader:** Darlene Rake; **Indexer:** Sharon Duffy; **Permission Manager:** Martha Gullo; **Graphic Designer:** Fred Starbird; **Graphic Artist:** Kathleen Boudreau-Fuoss; **Cover Designer:** Keith Blomberg; **Photo Asset Manager:** Laura Fitch; **Photo Production Manager:** Jason Allen; **Art Manager:** Kelly Hendren; **Illustrator and Associate Art Manager:** Alan L. Wilborn; **Printer:** United Graphics

Printed in the United States of America   10 9 8 7 6 5 4 3 2 1

The paper in this book is certified under a sustainable forestry program.

Human Kinetics
Web site: www.HumanKinetics.com

United States: Human Kinetics
P.O. Box 5076, Champaign, IL 61825-5076
800-747-4457
e-mail: humank@hkusa.com

Canada: Human Kinetics
475 Devonshire Road Unit 100,
Windsor, ON N8Y 2L5
800-465-7301 (in Canada only)
e-mail: info@hkcanada.com

Europe: Human Kinetics
107 Bradford Road, Stanningley,
Leeds LS28 6AT, United Kingdom
+44 (0) 113 255 5665
e-mail: hk@hkeurope.com

Australia: Human Kinetics
57A Price Avenue, Lower Mitcham,
South Australia 5062
08 8372 0999
e-mail: info@hkaustralia.com

New Zealand: Human Kinetics
Division of Sports Distributors NZ Ltd.
P.O. Box 300 226 Albany, North Shore City, Auckland
0064 9 448 1207
e-mail: info@humankinetics.co.nz

To those
who continually love
and support us

CONTENTS

PREFACE

Baby boomers, those born between 1946 and 1964, represent a generation that consists of nearly 76 million Americans. By the year 2011, the first wave of America's boomer generation will have turned 65 years of age. By that date, nearly all boomers will have entered or will be entering the life of retirement and leisure, bringing with them their varied life experiences, life values, and life expectations. All this will directly affect recreation and leisure professionals in terms of leisure programming and marketing.

Given the foreseen impact of the baby boomer generation, and given that recreation and leisure is a "demand-driven" profession, recreation professionals must be prepared to market and deliver a wide range of leisure opportunities that will serve a whole new set of demands. It appears that this will require a change in traditional attitudes about the needs and desires of older participants. No longer can it be assumed that bingo, art classes, and social dances will represent the collective leisure interests of retirees. In order to meet the leisure demands of boomers, recreation professionals will have to increasingly think in terms of active, vibrant participants rather than mere recipients of services. Over the next decade, the implications of this aging society will be significant for recreation professionals, making the planning, marketing, and delivery of leisure programs all the more challenging.

Recreation professionals and students need to fully understand the boomer generation in terms of culture, sociodemographics, values, and economics in order to make responsible future decisions regarding facilities, programs, services, and marketing techniques. If what is currently known about boomers holds true, it would seem logical for the recreation professional to recognize and understand differences in the makeup of the boomer generation from societal norms, and to strive to meet their demands through leisure programs and marketing efforts. If research is correct, boomers will be unlike any generation served in leisure today.

This reference book is written for the recreation professional, defined as someone who is involved in the process of planning, designing, marketing, and delivering leisure programs for baby boomers, and for the undergraduate university student, defined as someone who is studying for a bachelor's or similar degree in recreation, leisure, or tourism. The boomer population is the force behind the "changing" demographic picture of society today, and researchers have forecast their impact on the future (Gillon, 2004; Godbey, 2003; Parkel, 2003; Toffler, 1990). However, current research is lacking in fundamental information that is key to the recreation and leisure field with regard to working with boomers (Cochran, 2005).

Recreation professionals are busy; they want to locate information quickly and creatively. This book is organized in a reference format for ease of use. Target audience groups include university students in undergraduate or graduate recreation, tourism, or marketing programs and active professionals in the field of recreation and leisure who are involved in any sort of leisure programming and marketing with boomers. The authors currently work in the field: Their professional and personal expertise is reflected in the book's content and organization. This book gives you

- an in-depth review of current literature focused on the values of boomers;
- insight into and techniques for identifying the leisure interests of boomers;
- explanation and support for adopting a different philosophical lens, a "boomer lens," in order to succeed with this unique cohort;
- programming guidelines and program ideas for this population segment;
- ready-to-use marketing templates for leisure programming with boomers;
- insight into the future of boomers over the next decade and the foreseen aftereffect on leisure programming and marketing; and
- listings of books and Web sites to use as resources related to leisure programming and marketing.

The recreation profession exists to provide a service so that people's leisure experiences will be more meaningful and will have a positive impact upon quality of life. To measure their effectiveness against this objective, recreation professionals must recognize the diversity of the interests, lifestyles, and age groups they serve and must be able to program and market their services accordingly. Just as boomers demand and expect high-quality leisure opportunities, the recreation professional demands and deserves high-quality resources. It is our hope that this book will be a successful resource for leisure programming and marketing geared toward the baby boomer generation in your facilities, your parks, and your programs.

Chapter 1 sets a global picture of (a) who the baby boomers are and what makes them so different from previous cohorts, (b) the status of aging in our society, and (c) the impact that the baby boomer generation will have on the field of recreation and leisure over the next decade. With the support of current literature, including the research of one of the book's coauthors (Cochran, 2005), four value areas of boomers are reviewed in depth: cultural influences, social or lifestyle influences, retirement and leisure pursuits, and economics and education. These value areas set the stage for establishing the need for the leisure professional to pay attention to the coming wave of boomers.

Chapter 2 explains what drives boomers to leisure programs. The four value areas discussed in chapter 1 serve as the foundation for the Cochran Baby Boomer Quiz, which appears in the appendix. This tool fills a need unmet by currently available assessment tools. There are two versions of the Cochran Baby Boomer Quiz: one for boomers themselves and one for the recreation professional. The quiz allows examination of how values drive boomers to leisure programs, specifically competitive, educational, physiological, social, relaxation, and aesthetic values. The chapter uses the quiz as a foundation for understanding the values and philosphy in leisure regarding what boomers want. Recreation professionals can use this practical assessment with the boomers in their region to learn about their leisure values, and also use it with staff to assess their understanding of boomers.

Boomers have redefined every stage in their lives, and their impact on retirement and leisure will also be redefining. Marketing techniques that recreation professionals have employed in the past will not work for this population (Cochran, 2005). In order to effectively market leisure programs to the boomers, professionals need to understand more than just the boomer population itself. Chapter 3 presents an overview of the generations surrounding and including the boomers with regard to their demographic makeup, gender differences, cultural influences, consumer behavior and spending patterns, and brand loyalty, as well as the impact of generational values on various marketing tactics.

Marketing to boomers, instead of employing new perspectives, is currently conducted in the same way as leisure programming, relying on past practices and generalizations. Chapter 3 also presents ready-to-use marketing techniques that encompass boomer culture and values. Topics include the psychology of marketing; how to get boomers into recreation facilities and keep them in programs; advertising beyond use of the brochure; motivating, recruiting, and communicating at the front lines; and creating and maintaining a focused image.

The need for recreation professionals to adopt a different philosophical lens—a "boomer lens" that encompasses the values of this population—is essential to future success (Cochran, 2006). Chapter 4 presents insight into this notion and application through various examples. Using a boomer lens will allow the professional to (a) fully understand and create programs and marketing techniques that are responsive to an unusual aging society, (b) have an awareness of external opportunities and challenges that will foster innovation and a positive response to serving a new clientele of participants, and (c) consider specific value structures of this generation.

With bodies aging but spirits still strong, baby boomers are changing the face of recreation and leisure in many ways, which should drive programming beyond what our current senior centers offer (Cochran, 2005). The future of leisure programming and marketing with boomers presents unique opportunities that the recreation professional must not only know about but also proactively plan for and act upon. Additionally, chapter 4 presents a number of important guidelines that should help direct recreation professionals who are devising leisure programs, services, and marketing strategies for the baby boomer generation. This innovative set of guidelines consists of three main steps: (1) study the boomer picture; (2) assess your agency's preparedness; and (3) strategize for boomer programming, marketing, and implementation.

Resources available today focus on the mature adult—those over age 60—and do not take into account the values or the uniqueness of the boomer generation. Chapters 5 through 9 present in detail a variety of program areas and formats specific to the leisure program interests and values of the boomers, both today and during retirement, supported by current statistics and case studies. Chapter topics include arts and culture, education, outdoors and adventure, healthy lifestyles (fitness and sports), and tourism.

On January 1, 2011, the oldest members of the baby boomer generation will be turning 65 years of age. By that time the number of aging Americans will have skyrocketed. As boomers age, the look, meaning, experience, and purpose of maturity will be transformed. Because of this significant increase in the aging of our society and the fact that boomers are unlike any other generation, it is imperative that the recreation professional be prepared to provide leisure programs and create marketing schemes appropriate to this population. Chapter 10 projects the implications of boomers in the future with respect to (a) the field of recreation and leisure as a whole, (b) impacts on marketing trends, and (c) ways in which professionals can prepare for what will happen after the boomers.

In the appendix you will find two tools, Cochran Baby Boomer Quizzes 1 and 2, that are ready for your use in assessing boomers and in evaluating recreation professional expertise regarding leisure programming for this dynamic cohort.

1

Are You Ready for the Boomers?

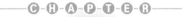

The impact of America's 76 million baby boomers on our leisure facilities and in our programs is going to be profound. In order to accommodate this significant population and their leisure needs, recreation professionals must realize that the current practices in leisure programming will be challenged with this age group in terms of how programs are designed and delivered to an aging, dynamic, and active population.

As recreation professionals, we provide myriad programs to all walks of life; and our success relies not only on an understanding of what our participants like to do, but also on an understanding of what makes them who they are—whether they are children, teenagers, young adults, or seniors. Today we are faced with the challenge, or to some the opportunity, to provide leisure programs for a dynamic and demanding group, the baby boomers. We hear this name over and over again as boomers have gained the attention of demographers, politicians, marketers, and social scientists over the last 60 years and will continue to do so for the next 25 years. Many recreation professionals today are boomers themselves; on the other hand, many are not, creating a more challenging environment in terms of leisure programming and marketing for a generation that is not their own. This chapter is designed to set a global picture of who the boomers are and the impact that boomers will have in the field of recreation and leisure. It is with this information that we can begin to form a basis for leisure programming and marketing with boomers.

WHO ARE THE BOOMERS?

The return in 1946 of millions of World War II soldiers from battlefields and military units, combined with the desire of married couples to start a family, resulted in the largest generation born in history, the baby boomer generation. In the United States, nearly 76 million children were born from 1946 to 1964. In Canada, there were 9.8 million births during this same time period (Most, 1996). Similar birth rates occurred in Europe and Asia coinciding with the end of World War II. Other explanations for the baby boom include the positive economic climate, the changing social values of postwar society, and the acceptance of large family size and status. Reasons for the end of the baby boom in the mid-1960s are harder to pinpoint. Factors often cited include expanded educational opportunities for young women, which encouraged them to defer marriage and child-rearing; increased participation of females in the workplace; and the widespread availability of oral contraceptives and other birth control methods. Current literature reveals four areas that set the stage for understanding boomers: cultural influences, lifestyle, retirement and leisure pursuits, and economics and education.

Cultural Influences

Baby boomers appear to have a perception of themselves as very different from other generations: a perception that has existed since childhood and has to do largely with attitude, lifestyle, social roles, and political values. Sociologically, boomers are said to be defined by shared values and history; their parents lived through the Great Depression and World War II, and boomers were influenced by the ideals fostered during those events.

The boomer generation see themselves as the beneficiaries of progress. They were raised in a period of unprecedented prosperity and unparalleled expectations of the future (Gillon, 2004). As a whole, boomers have participated in a variety of life experiences from the Cold War to Vietnam, the civil rights and women's movements, and a sexual revolution; their experience included the arrival of Elvis, the Beach Boys, hula hoops, the Mickey Mouse Club, home freezers, television, minivans, and a pop culture that speaks for itself. Their distinct attitudes have been shown through their continual lifestyle of free choice, their uninhibited search for what looks and feels right, and a desire to do things differently than their parents' generation did (Dychtwald, 1999).

Though 18 years may span the baby boomer generation as a whole, it should be noted that there is a distinct difference between the younger and older boomers. In general, the baby boomers born between 1946 and 1955 have a different outlook on life than those born between 1956 and 1964. The oldest of the boomers were heavily influenced by countercultural events such as the assassinations of John F. Kennedy, Robert Kennedy, and Martin Luther King; political unrest; the walk on the moon; the Vietnam War; antiwar protests; social experimentation; sexual freedom; the civil rights movement; the environmental movement; the women's movement; protests and riots; and experimentation with various intoxicating recreational substances. Their attitudes are characterized by descriptors such as "experimental," "individualism," and "free spirited" and are oriented toward social causes.

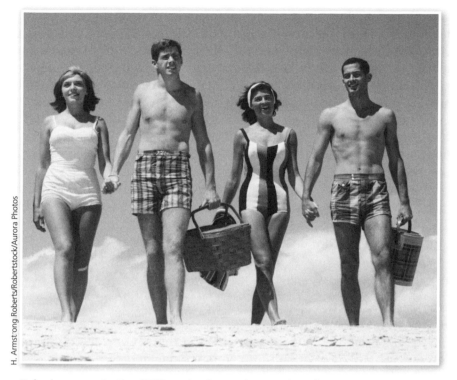

H. Armstrong Roberts/Robertstock/Aurora Photos

Baby boomers in the 1960s—check out those swimsuits!

On the other hand, the second group, born between 1956 and 1964, was more influenced by memorable events such as Watergate, Nixon's resignation, the Cold War, the oil embargo, raging inflation, and gasoline shortages. Their attitudes are characterized by the phrases "less optimistic," "distrust of government," and "general cynicism," resulting in a practical and balance-seeking approach to life. Together, baby boomers are the children of the first large-scale middle class in history. Not only are the boomers 76 million strong, but they so influenced American culture that *Time* magazine in 1966 broke with tradition and selected the baby boomer generation instead of an individual as its "Man of the Year."

Increasingly importantly, boomers are said to be most readily distinguished from previous generations by their personal values. They appear to be open-minded about a wide range of political notions; however, they are also deeply patriotic, think for themselves, and are rarely hesitant to voice their opinions. With regard to economic issues, 51 percent of boomers in the United States are apt to describe themselves as more conservative than some may have thought, yet continue to consider themselves quite socially liberal (Keating, 2004). The issue of free choice appears to be important as boomers continue to be pro-choice on the abortion issue, believe in the Equal Rights Amendment, and want flexible work schedules and child care for their families. Based on the sheer number of boomers, it is estimated that the boomer generation will hold a plurality in Congress until 2015 and in the White House until 2021, and that they will have a majority in the Supreme Court from 2010 to 2030—therefore making up the vast majority of the political, cultural, industrial, and academic leadership class in the United States.

Baby boomers have made statements in music, fashion, education, women's rights, television, advertising, technology, and medicine. Boomers defined rock 'n' roll with legends such as Linda Ronstadt, Ozzy Osbourne, Bruce Springsteen, Billy Joel, the Rolling Stones, and Madonna, to name a few. The Vietnam conflict, the draft, and military deferment—for those enrolled in a university program—kept many baby boom males in institutions of higher learning. In addition, the desire for equality propelled many women of baby boomer age into higher education, resulting in the most highly educated, influential, and prosperous generation in U.S. history. Society will be influenced by this dominance until it literally dies away.

Lifestyle

It is no secret that America is aging. Newspapers, television, magazines, government, and scholarly reports tell us that the first wave of the baby boomer generation are now entering their retirement years and that we are on the threshold of a major shift in demographic characteristics. In the next 30 years our nation's "senior" population will double due to the sheer size of the boomer generation; and thanks to medical and health advancements, boomers will live longer than any previous generation.

With such a large increase in births over a defined period of time, the baby boomer generation has importantly influenced the character of the U.S. population. Boomers have created an unprecedented population explosion, with the oldest of this generation turning 62 this year; by 2030 all surviving baby boomers will be between the ages of 66 and 84. According to the U.S. Census Bureau (2000), in the year 2005, 42 percent of boomers were over the age of 50 years. Further, America's boomers make up 27.5 percent of the population, having an estimated annual spending power of $2.1 trillion, and compose 45.8 million households with average spending of $46,000 per household (CBS News, 2006).

Today, the median age of the U.S. population has risen to its highest point in history. The current average age for men is 34.7 years and for women 37.4 years, with the median age of the U.S. population at 36 years of age (World Factbook, 2004). By the year 2050, the projected median age will be 41. Moreover, the Administration on Aging (2002) projects that the over-50 age group will grow from about 13 percent of the total population in 2000 to 20 percent in 2030 and remain above 20 percent for at least several decades thereafter. Likewise, the Bureau's population projection shows that 18 million persons will be age 85 or older in 2050 (4-1/2 percent of the U.S. population) or, simply put, that one in five Americans will be ages 65 years and older. This clearly reflects how boomers will affect our aging society.

Though aging is inevitable, boomers have continually had an obsession with fitness, another main identifying characteristic of this generation. A significant number of boomers have proven to be more physically active than those in previous generations. This is shown in the number of increased health club memberships for those aged 55 years and older over the past 12 years (Meisler, 2003) and active participation in a variety of fitness events. Boomers are said to feel that they will live longer than prior generations as they are already implementing a healthy lifestyle within their retirement plans—for example through exercise and positive eating habits—and they continue to feel several years younger than their actual age. A recent study by the American Association of Retired Persons (AARP, 2004) supported this notion; the results showed that the mean age among baby boomers was 47, but the mean age that they felt was 40.

For the recreation professional, this means that boomers are going to be the most active seniors who have ever lived. One thing is for sure: They are intent on feeling youthful and not allowing the aging process to affect their life negatively, though some take a critical view of their attempts to maintain their youth through yoga, plastic surgery, and Viagra. Despite what others may say, boomers do not recognize limits and envision themselves well into their 70s doing in-line skating, running marathons, riding Harley-Davidsons, climbing the world's highest peaks, and taking on wild endeavors (Cochran, 2005)—showing society that, as this group may age, their diversity grows increasingly clearer.

Retirement and Leisure Pursuits

As the baby boomer generation enters midlife, a new set of social and economic factors is beginning to influence their leisure time and activities. Boomers

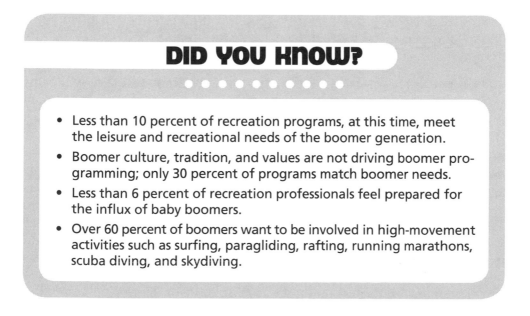

DID YOU KNOW?

- Less than 10 percent of recreation programs, at this time, meet the leisure and recreational needs of the boomer generation.
- Boomer culture, tradition, and values are not driving boomer programming; only 30 percent of programs match boomer needs.
- Less than 6 percent of recreation professionals feel prepared for the influx of baby boomers.
- Over 60 percent of boomers want to be involved in high-movement activities such as surfing, paragliding, rafting, running marathons, scuba diving, and skydiving.

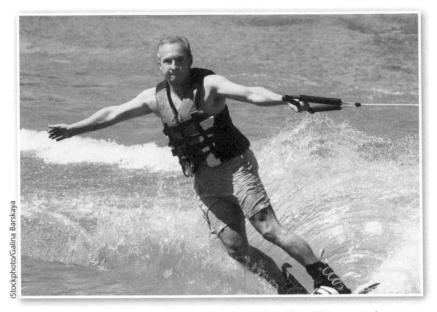

Retirement no longer conjures up images of golf and bingo. Baby boomers continue to be adventure-seekers, even in their golden years.

know what they want from retirement. As a group in general, boomers are known to work hard, play hard, and spend hard (Ziegler, 2002). They are looking for a lively and entertaining experience during retirement. It is said that boomers will use leisure opportunities to search for balance, lasting relationships, and spiritual values, in addition to treating leisure as a necessity (Belsie, 2001). Their attitudes can be attributed to their sense of adventure, "breaking" the rules, doing things differently from how people did them in the past.

We can recognize boomer attitude as leisure continues to factor into boomers' expectations for retirement. An AARP report (2004) supports this notion:

- 70 percent of boomers have a hobby or special interest they will dedicate more time to.
- 68 percent agree they will have more time for recreation during retirement.
- 51 percent expect to volunteer and devote more time to community service.

If boomers hold true to form, they are also likely to spend the vast percentage of their assets on travel and leisure (Updegrave, 2004).

It is well known that Sun City, founded by Del Webb Corporation in the 1960s, was the first residential development to serve as a destination of glorified leisure and the chance for endless play. Here a leisured lifestyle became the ideal for success in later life. Marketers suggest that boomers have a renewed interest in leisure and entertainment as they have outgrown the materialism of the '80s and are focusing more on home and family life

(Elias, 2001). This may be reflected in gardening, cooking, do-it-yourself home improvements, and other serenity-oriented activities.

In contrast, many boomers appear to be interested in remaining in their own homes for the rest of their lives. Recent data from the U.S. Census Bureau show that though many boomers consider moving to sunshine states, they are now remaining in their current location or relocating to Northwest and East Coast areas that are closer to their families. This gives boomers opportunities for community involvement, entertaining education, and civic engagement through their local community level, as well as the opportunity to fulfill their active lifestyles in fitness and recreation. For many, retirement will become a cyclical blend of work, education, and leisure.

If boomers choose to reside in retirement communities, they will be demanding high-tech fitness centers, active recreational pursuits, diverse cultural programs, extensive walking trails, and university courses that are taught on-site (Todd, 2004). Did you know that golf is no longer the mainstay feature of retirement communities? Boomers will be influencing a shift in thinking with an emphasis on leisure not just as a means of relaxation or play, but also as a means for continued growth (Dychtwald & Flower, 1992). It is predicted that maintaining an active lifestyle will be fundamental to boomers as they enter retirement. Marketers will argue that this group will generally not tolerate stereotypes or ageism. Most boomers will be striving to maintain their youth physically and mentally and view retirement as an active period in their lives; they will expect stylish products to instill value beyond mere utility. Boomers will not go quietly into retirement; they want high-quality experiences and have the discretionary income to support their desires.

As their lives have indicated thus far, it would appear that the boomer generation will demand more than what our current senior centers and retirement communities are providing. It is speculated that these facilities "simply are not going to unleash the talent or capture the imagination as this dominant population enters the next stage of their lives" (Freedman, 1999, p. 22). If what we know about boomers is true, the traditional senior center will have to break out of its isolation to meet the demands of the baby boomer generation. Therefore, senior centers will be compelled to develop a large range and scope of adult-focused recreational activities targeted at a program philosophy that entails the psychological, educational, physiological, social, and demographic interests of this cohort. It would seem logical for the recreation professional to recognize these demands and meet them. Consequentially, every industry providing leisure services will be affected by the aging baby boomer generation.

Economics and Education

Baby boomers in general have done better than any previous generation in terms of income and education, resulting in better overall life satisfaction

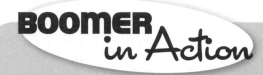

Debbie Dickerson

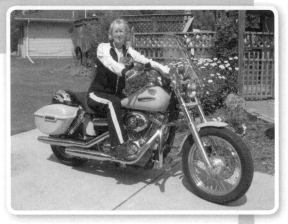

"You will never catch me riding a motorcycle!" That would have been my response had the question been posed to me a few years ago. But something happens when your children are grown and you realize that you're suddenly on the fast track of middle age. When my brother approached (okay, nagged) my husband and me to just take the rider safety class to see if I liked it, I reluctantly agreed. Having never even driven a stick shift before, I was scared to death at that first class. At the end of the class when I passed the written exam with flying colors and by some miracle passed the driving test (having never once dropped the bike!), I was hooked and cautiously began my motorcycling hobby.

I began practicing a little at a time in parking lots, and today I take long rides on the open road, enjoying the total sensory experience of the changing seasons in the Midwest. So, at 50-something, I am still chasing after my older brothers, in a Harley kind of way! Oh, and don't even ask them whose bike has the biggest motor and six speeds—my "bike boys" will turn green with envy. No tattoos, of course, but my wardrobe has expanded to include the most stylish biker wear. I now mentor other lady motorcycle enthusiasts, cheering them on as they take their first tentative rides.

I'm a succession planning analyst for a Fortune 100 company in corporate America, so my colleagues are quite surprised by my unusual hobby. My family and friends are concerned for my safety and sanity. To all I say this: Life is an open road. Ride on! Ride free!

Profile and photo courtesy of Debbie Dickerson.

(Gillon, 2004). According to the fourth national survey of baby boomers conducted by Del Webb Corporation, the median household income is 35 to 53 percent higher than that of their parents' generation, and about 25 to 30 percent of U.S. baby boomers have four or more years of college education

than generations before them ("Leading Edge Baby Boomers," 2001). Women of the boomer generation want both careers and families whereas men want to equal the achievements of their parents. The income and educational leverage of this group translates into opportunities and expectations of retirement that could not be realized previously by society. However, according to U.S. Census data (2000), approximately 57 million boomers, roughly 70 percent, came from poor, working-class, or family-business backgrounds.

The impact of baby boomers on the workforce is noticeable in the labor force median age. When boomers entered the workforce, the median age of the labor force decreased; as they aged, the median age of the labor force increased. By 2025, the workforce will be older, with 40 percent of workers age 45 and over compared to 33 percent in 1998 (Bayer & Bonilla, 2001). The Bureau of Labor Statistics predicts that the number of workers 55 and older will jump 4 percent annually, making them the fastest-growing age group.

While a number of studies have shown that most boomers are not saving nearly enough for their retirement, others have reached much more optimistic conclusions. The average household income today for baby boomers ranges from $56,500 to $58,889 before taxes ("Demographic Profile," 2003), giving them the highest median household incomes in the United States.

Research conducted by AARP (2004) projects that most baby boomers will be retired in 2030 and will receive Social Security benefits along with pension and asset income. Therefore, boomers will have a higher economic status than their parents' generation had at the same ages. Despite these positive predictions, the need for boomers to work during retirement for supplementary income is increasing. Up to 80 percent of boomers in the United States plan to start new careers or continue former careers but in a different fashion.

Boomers have redefined the concepts of youth, early adulthood, and middle age, so it's safe to say that they'll recast retirement. Boomers are demanding; they expect value for their money; they want quality products, and they expect convenience. The total number of people age 65 and over will significantly increase, adding importance to the need for recreation professionals to understand how to devise adequate leisure programs and appropriate marketing avenues for this unique cohort.

THE BOOMER EFFECT ON RECREATION AND LEISURE

The recreation professional of today, whether involved in a municipal, private, nonprofit, or tourism organization, is concerned with the many and varied ideas about recreation and leisure. Recreation professionals are increasingly faced with the need to develop a variety of experiences to suit their participants. Recreation and leisure programs encompass a wide variety of sports and games, travel and tourism, hobbies and the arts, entertainment, fitness pursuits, social activities, and outdoor recreation. The opportunities for leisure services are unlimited, and vary from programs for individuals to public or private services for corporations and government entities on land and at sea. A major concern for professionals in recreation is the vast scope of the opportunities, making it frustrating sometimes to decide what should have the highest priority, especially when resources and economics are limited.

As the population is dramatically increasing in age, recreation professionals need to be aware of the significance of this phenomenon. Baby boomers are currently a dominant contributor to our aging society, and there are indications that they are not going to be the traditional senior. Boomers cannot be compiled into one category and be called senior citizens, though they may legally be of senior citizen age (Ziegler & O'Sullivan, 2004). This categorization is currently common among recreation practitioners and members of society as they struggle to find a place for baby boomers.

We must further consider that leisure behavior and preferences of boomers will be based on their health status, the amount of available discretionary income, and lifestyle. There will be different needs and expectations from the older to the younger generation of baby boomers. Merging learning and travel in the form of adventure vacations is assumed to hold promising opportunities for both public and private leisure providers ("Active Vacations," 2003). Most boomers are doers, not sitters. Further, adults between the ages of 39 and 58 (roughly the range of the boomer population) are 6 percent more likely than the national average to be involved in some type of sporting activity (Fetto, 2000).

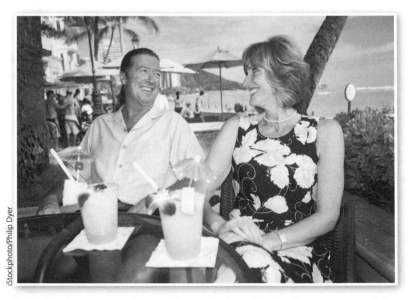

Baby boomers stay young at heart by keeping in close contact with their friends. Laughing and socializing are also great ways to relieve stress.

Boomers have different expectations, are more self-indulgent, do not seem concerned with added costs of leisure services, will aim to volunteer, and will be able to create things that work for them during retirement. Boomers enjoy individualized activities rather than group events and also like socializing within small groups or extended family circles (Todd, 2004). Additionally, equipment and services that are consistent with an active, recreation-oriented lifestyle will be forced not only to expand but also to accommodate the diverse interests of the new baby boomer participants. This includes consideration of facility scheduling, program offerings, equipment, marketing techniques, and participant attitudes.

Recreation and leisure is not limited to providing parks, programs, or facilities. It involves the dedication of community members to its mission. Therefore, it should be expected that the sheer number of boomers, combined with their desire for leisure, will lead increasingly to expanding representation on recreation councils, commissions, and advisory boards and in professional organizations. Moreover, their political influence will affect policies and programs designed with interests of older adults in mind.

The government, the church, the military, the professions, and the schools have all been reformed in one way or another by the baby boomers. Baby boomers will be satisfied not simply with an affluent society; they will be satisfied only with one that will fulfill the expectations fostered by their self-confidence and sophistication. Peter Drucker, a leader in 20th-century business organization, has said, "The best way to predict the future is to create it" (O'Sullivan, 2004). Just as baby boomers have done in society throughout their lives, this is what leisure professionals must do to meet the needs of boomers.

The boomer generation is looking for consistent delivery of a unique experience. In order to provide this experience, the recreation professional must be prepared to deliver a wide range of leisure opportunities and to serve a whole new set of demands created by the boomer generation. It would appear that this will require a change in traditional attitudes about the needs and desires of older participants. No longer can it be assumed that bingo, art classes, and social dances will represent the collective leisure interests of the baby boomers in retirement. It appears that in the future, recreation professionals will have to increasingly think in terms of active, vibrant participants rather than mere recipients of services. In addition, leisure services and experiences once considered appropriate only for younger adults may increasingly be sought by the "new" generation of retirees (Cochran, 2005). Thus it is argued that the nonmoral good that comes from leisure services must be distributed to all individuals, especially the boomers, in an appropriate manner. The future of leisure for the baby boomers thus begins with examining existing leisure programming practices and proceeds to developing a different leisure programming philosophy for this active, educated, and unique cohort.

What Drives Boomers?

Boomers have left everlasting marks on society. They have extensively influenced the education system, growth and marketing within the economy, and the emergence of alternative lifestyles, as well as contributing to dramatic shifts in the nature and structure of families. The importance of recreation and leisure in their lives is another significant change. As we know, leisure can be a meaningful alternative to work as well as provide an opportunity for important interaction with significant others; it is also crucial for one's self-concept and sense of well-being. Though some may choose to work for financial or social reasons, the majority of boomers appear to be preparing for retirement as a time of leisure. Boomers appear to realize that work may have provided their income but that what enhances their personal well-being is the experiences derived during leisure. For this reason, it is safe to say that boomers will be looking to leisure providers—you—to offer them an array of programs and services that will distinguish them from previous generations, primarily based on their value structure.

WHAT BOOMERS WANT

As we discussed in chapter 1, compared to previous middle-aged generations, boomers have a higher occupational status, resulting in more discretionary income; and due to their focus on defying the aging process, they have improved health in their later years. From a leisure programming perspective, this means that we will need to anticipate the growing demands for recreational resources used by physically fit, financially aware, health-conscious consumers who happen to be of retirement age. In order to do so, we must understand what drives boomers to participate in our leisure programs.

The Nature of Boomer Programming

At the simplest level, leisure programming is the process of providing opportunities for recreational participation, including activities such as sports, games, hobbies, fitness classes, arts and crafts, music, drama, and dance, or social events as seen in most community parks and recreation program guides. Leisure programming refers to the entire comprehensive set of programs that an agency offers and not just to one specific leisure experience. We can say that being a good leisure programmer involves the ability to systematically identify and meet the leisure needs and interests of various participant age groups and ability levels. We can also say that the participant, through the use of leisure programs, forms values, develops skills, and learns processes of recreation and leisure (Edginton et al., 2004). As recreation professionals, we must remember that leisure programs are not an end in themselves; responding to the needs and desires of our participants is the true reason for the existence of leisure service agencies. Therefore, it is important to keep in mind that our participants are the focal point of leisure programs and services.

We know that leisure is an important element in the lives of most people and that the term "leisure" has different meanings to different people under different circumstances. As with many aspects of the broad field of recreation and leisure, there is no simple definition that has meaning for everyone.

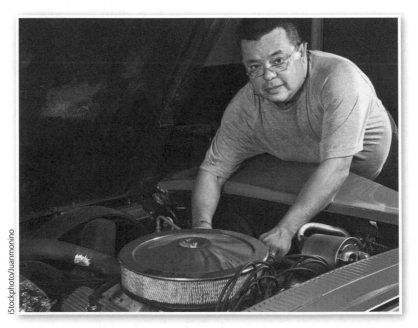

Baby boomers enjoy a wide range of hobbies. They like to work with their hands and spend time on projects that are meaningful to them. It's very satisfying to see a challenging project through to completion, such as fixing up an antique car.

Boomers value freedom, and leisure is an expression of that freedom. There is no one way of planning or conducting leisure programming. Traditionally leisure programming has been implemented using a number of different program approaches or theories. Theory may be defined as a principle or collection of principles that possibly explain some behavior, as a means to clarify the relationship between a particular proposition, as statements linking abstract concepts to empirical data, and as premises to account for data (Rudestam & Newton, 2001). Understanding leisure theory allows a recreation programmer to better understand the meaning or purpose of the participants' leisure activity choices or involvement in order to create environments in which these experiences can occur. Such knowledge gives us a conceptual framework for understanding leisure behavior and providing leisure activities or services—with the end result that we can provide adequately for the boomer generation. Regardless of which programming approach we use, it has to apply to our target audience. The following are common program theories aimed at describing various approaches to providing leisure programs and services (Cochran, 2005; Edginton et al., 2004):

1. Traditional approach: Builds primarily on the basis of what has been done in the past, with the idea that what has been done in the past has been popular and successful and should be continued.

2. Current practices approach: Relies heavily on copying what is being done in other communities, including adopting new fads, to understand programming needs—for example, following practices that are highlighted in professional literature, featured in presentations at conferences, and observed in programs elsewhere.

3. Expressed-desires approach: Relies on surveys, interviews, or interest checklists that indicate what participants would like to have offered in leisure programs. The assumption is that their expressed wishes will heavily influence the selection of program activities to be offered.

4. Cafeteria approach: Makes a large selection of varied offerings available to the potential participant, who is able to select the activity that seems most appealing based on free choice.

5. Benefits-based approach: Focuses on sharply defining the benefits and positive outcomes of leisure programs by taking a more developmental approach to planning.

Though there may be different approaches to and theories on cultivating leisure experiences, philosophically leisure has been taught as a means to understand the concept of leisure as a whole.

Plato and Aristotle saw leisure as a product of selective disengagement, relaxation, contemplation, and private enjoyment (Kleiber, 1985). Leisure has also been described as the basis of culture in that celebration and affirmation ensure its continuance and the ritualization of playfulness offers new cultural forms (Pieper, 1965). The study of leisure has primarily evolved into three basic approaches, relating to time, activity, and state of mind (Godbey, 2003). According to some research (deGrazia, 1964), relative freedom from obligation is traditionally regarded as the essence of leisure; another view (Neulinger, 1974) holds that it is possible for people to be at leisure even when at work. Other leisure scholars have focused on leisure as a state of mind or attitude, either transitorily or as a way of life (Csikszentmihalyi, 1990; Iso-Ahola & Mannell, 1985).

When we synthesize all of these approaches or theories, we come much closer to a philosophic, definitive explanation of leisure behavior that may help us design and implement leisure programs and services. Usually we use these philosophic approaches very pragmatically and practically. Leisure programming typically begins with cursory knowledge about a group of leisure participants; or, if we are using a specific program approach, we tend to collect general information rather than specific, individual information. This chapter focuses primarily on the reasoning behind the use of a philosophical approach to leisure programming, one that is significant for the application of leisure programs and services. Unless we provide meaningful activities, boomers will become bored.

Why Philosophy in Boomer Programming?

Philosophy does not necessarily generate new knowledge; but it is the nexus of our culture and our value systems, which we formally study through epistemology, ethics, politics, and even aesthetics. Philosophy raises questions about what we do and why we do it, and goes beyond individual cases and phenomena to treat questions of a general nature. Philosophy is a more reflective and systematic activity than common sense, and its power for recreation professionals lies in its ability to help them better understand and appreciate the activities of everyday life (Elias & Merriam, 1995). But how can we use such an abstract definition and apply it to a useful service such as leisure programming? To begin, we can use philosophy to answer a series of meaningful philosophical questions:

- Is our present approach to leisure programming capturing the true essence of individual, specific information about our clients' leisure interests?
- Is our approach helping us understand personal, objective, and subjective values about leisure?
- We may capture the objective information through a check sheet, but would we know more about wants and needs if we could capture the subjective nature of needs and wants?

For example, an objective value might be expressed by the statement "I swim because I want to get fit"; the subjective value might be expressed by the statements "I swim because I enjoy my body moving through water," or "I find meaning in my life through exercise and swimming." These subjective values are not easy to capture, but we argue that they *can* be captured and that practical philosophy might help us answer these important questions (Charles, 2002; Kretchmar, 2000). Without using a philosophical approach to leisure programming on a regular basis, recreation professionals may not adequately meet the needs of diverse populations, nor will participants receive the quality of leisure that they desire and deserve. Understanding leisure values and leisure needs is necessary to an effective philosophical approach to boomer programming.

> **If you don't like the road you're walking, start paving another one.**
> —*Dolly Parton*

Understanding Leisure Values

When something is important to us, when it is viewed as worthwhile, desirable, or consequential, such a thing is said to have value. Values permeate society and influence all aspects of life. They can be viewed from a societal, group, or individual perspective. Your values (beliefs or attitudes about what is good, right, desirable, worthwhile, and so on) and your value system (the ways you organize, rank, and prioritize things for making decisions based on your values) provide the foundation for your personal and professional judgments and choices. They are your beliefs about what is important in life. Some values refer to how one should act (for example, to be honest, self-disciplined, kind). Other values refer to what one wants to accomplish or what one wants to obtain in life (for example, a lot of money, security, fame, health, salvation, wisdom).

Your values exist as a complex set of interweaving personal policies or priorities that serve as a guide for decision making. Values may be based on knowledge, aesthetic considerations, practicality, moral grounds, or a combination of these. Much of what we value is not concerned with our sense of morality or ethics, so not all values can be called moral ones. Most of us value money, status, personal fulfillment, freedom, and world peace; and while these are not immoral values, they are not necessarily moral values.

When values relate specifically to leisure or leisure activities, they can be referred to as leisure nonmoral values. Leisure nonmoral values play an important role in determining how we view leisure and the types of activities we choose to participate in. When looking at nonmoral leisure values, we are considering those abstract categories associated with leisure about which we have strong feelings. In selecting leisure activities, some people place value on feelings of excitement, some place value on perceptual freedom, some value self-expression, and others value personal growth. These in turn are a reflection of attitudes that support these nonmoral values. Examples are the social benefits of leisure, or the physical fitness that is accrued from the activity, or even the feeling of general goodwill derived from engaging in leisure activities (Kretchmar, 2004).

As we have already emphasized, the baby boomer generation is a different generation than any other. Baby boomers have been labeled by society all their lives. They are unique with regard to their pop culture, their values, and their beliefs; and they are healthier, wealthier, and more highly educated than any other generation. Boomers are movers and shakers. They are a dynamic generation that will not take leisure, retirement, or aging lying down; they stand on the opposite end of the spectrum from lying down. Providing recreation programs should be based on understanding the participants, in terms of not only who they are but what they like to do, when they like to do it, and how they like to do it. In other words, programs should be based on the values of the given cohort.

Even though this book is centered on the concept of values driving leisure programming and marketing, some social-psychological researchers have argued that participation is driven by leisure needs. Therefore, we also need to understand the concept of leisure needs.

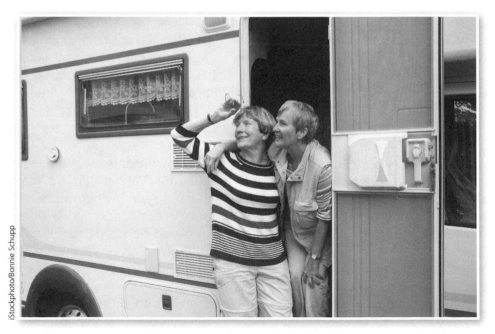

iStockphoto/Bonnie Schupp

Social interaction is vitally important for people of all ages. People are healthier and more active when they have solid support from peers.

Leisure Needs

Needs and values are obviously closely related. However, needs are described differently by a philosopher and a social psychologist. The philosopher focuses on the abstract value, whereas the social psychologist focuses on what is perceived to be a psychological process. The philosopher would argue that values come before needs; the social psychologist may not agree. In order to completely understand leisure programming with boomers, we need to consider social psychological needs. For example, social psychologists argue that we place great value on those things that we need in order to survive. Relating more to leisure, several studies indicate that most human beings have a strong need for affiliation with other people. Iso-Ahola (1980) argues that when people's circumstances isolate them from others, it is likely that leisure activities meeting the need for social interaction will dominate over other needs.

A BOOMER VALUE APPROACH

We need to keep in mind that much of what we think we know about senior recreation nonmoral values today will be redefined under the boomer generation; a wide range of opportunities awaits recreation professionals who anticipate the leisure challenges of the boomer cohort. With respect to the future of leisure programming with baby boomers, certain nonmoral values related to their retirement and aging are continually emerging and are supported by current literature. Chapter 1 presented information in four areas based on these emerging values; accordingly, the foundation of philosophy and values in this book consists of culture, lifestyle, retirement and leisure pursuits, and economic and educational values. If we develop and implement programs for this cohort based on elements other than those dominant in current literature, we as recreation professionals are failing to understand the true nature of this cohort and the potential for leisure derived from their values:

1. Culture: Boomers have rallied together regardless of the issue, have rebelled against authority, and have done things that made them feel good. They have an ability to deal with change but also to create situations demanding of social change. Their unique personalities come from a time in society when limits were imposed on how to live their lives. This will continue until they die.

2. Lifestyle: Having led America's health revolution, boomers are physically capable of working and producing much later in life than any previous generation simply because they've taken care of themselves and will continue to do so into the next phase of their lives. Thus, the value of healthy aging and its effect on society constitute an important trend.

3. Retirement and leisure pursuits: Retirement is not a signal for the end of a work life but rather a chance to pursue interests, change careers, or start a new business. It is often said that boomers want high-quality experiences and have the discretionary income to support their desires. Thus, their pursuits and the values placed on these pursuits will be radically different from those of past generations.

4. Economic and educational values: Boomers are the first generation to have been universally educated, given unprecedented access to higher education, and raised in a period of unmatched prosperity; and they have incomparable expectations about the future. Because of these elements, it is necessary to understand how this history of prosperity and educational attainment feeds into the boomers' values about leisure.

The success of a recreation program, the management of an agency, and the availability of a recreation facility or park service, combined with the foresight of recreation professionals, are all secrets to success. Recreation professionals need to recognize that baby boomers do not have the same interests or nonmoral leisure values as our current senior population. Knowing that many of the boomers are on their way to retirement, if not already there, we must take a proactive approach to the development and implementation of leisure programs, services, and facilities for this new cohort—one that encompasses their nonmoral values and uses a different philosophical lens to get to know boomers through their nonmoral values. In other words, recreation professionals cannot provide adequate programs, facilities, or services if they do not understand the population being served and are not able to foresee the direction in which their agency may be headed. One way to prepare is through use of a boomer assessment, as reflected in the Cochran Baby Boomer Quiz.

Assess Your Baby Boomer Knowledge

As you become familiar with the literature and consider the four nonmoral values that have emerged, you might wonder if all the information promulgated about boomers is correct. Another question you may have is whether the boomers as a group actually play out these values. If they do, to what extent are recreation programmers knowledgeable about this cohort? These questions lead to the idea of assessment.

Taking into account what is known about the baby boomers, recreation professionals will need to consider how to gather information about this population in a "fun" way—because fun is important to this new cohort, and the baby boomers are said to balk at the status quo way of collecting data (Cochran, 2005). Given the need for leisure programming to encompass a different focus, one that uses philosophy, it is appropriate for recreation professionals to use an assessment tool that captures the nonmoral values of the baby boomer cohort and also evaluates their own boomer readiness levels. In the remaining sections of the chapter we discuss the Cochran Baby Boomer Quiz and how you can use it to assess the needs of boomers in your community. These tools are designed for your adaptation and use (see appendix).

The Cochran Baby Boomer Quiz (CBBQ)

In the year 2011, the first wave of America's baby boomer generation will have turned 65 years of age. By this date, nearly all of the 76 million boomers will have entered or will be entering the life of retirement and leisure. They will continue to redefine the next phase of their lives as they have done in the past. The effect on the future of leisure programming will be profound. In assessing leisure interests, leisure programmers typically use the same set of survey questions that has been used for various populations rather than gearing survey questions toward the specific values of the population of interest. As a result, they are faced with issues such as low program sign-ups and poor retention rates.

An active research study on this issue (Cochran, 2005), which involved examining the literature on boomers and studying boomers themselves, showed that boomers revolted from a traditional survey. In initial pilot studies using common programming questions, the boomers refused to answer the typical questions. Using a different assessment based on the boomers' values of fun and education made it possible to learn much more about their values and about what drives their participation in leisure activities (see Cochran Baby Boomer Quizzes 1 and 2 in the appendix). Results indicated that as had been presumed, boomers have strong values in terms of their culture, impact on society, unique leisure and retirement perspectives, and economics.

What Professionals Know

Both boomers and recreation professionals took the quiz. Responses to the first 26 multiple-choice questions (see appendix), drawn from current literature and encompassing four distinct nonmoral values that make boomers who they are (culture, social, retirement and leisure pursuits, and economic and educational values), indicated that although baby boomers and recreation professionals responded similarly in some ways, there were noteworthy differences:

1. Boomer culture: The responses of the two groups to questions about culture were similar, indicating that yes, what society says about boomers is true—who they are, what influences them, and how they changed society.

2. Lifestyle: Recreation professionals were aware of the impact that boomers will have on society as a whole cohort; however, they did not know what percent of boomers were over the age of 50 in the year 2005. Boomers were not aware of the sheer size of their group within society and did not know their current ages. For both recreation professionals and boomers, these gaps may be due to poor mathematics, lack of common knowledge, or lack of awareness of the significance of this type of information.

3. Retirement and leisure pursuits: With respect to retirement activities, though boomers were interested in golf, it was not a priority in their choice of leisure activities. On the other hand, many recreation professionals felt that golf might still be a major activity for boomers during retirement. This discrepancy points to the need for recreation professionals to understand the leisure activities that drive boomers in order to effectively provide leisure programs or facilities during their retirement. Regarding leisure pursuit values, both participant groups had a strong understanding of the nonmoral leisure values of boomers. However, both groups failed to realize the dynamics within leisure formats that boomers choose to participate in, that is, individually or within smaller groups. Recognizing the dynamics of leisure participation allows the recreation professional to provide successful leisure programs and promotes high boomer participation levels.

4. Economic and education values: Neither boomers nor recreation professionals identified the median income level of this age group per individual as shown by research ($50,000-$60,000); both groups identified the median income level as either higher or lower. However, boomers and recreation professionals responded differently to questions about how boomers would spend their money in the future. While boomers' responses indicated that they would spend their money on leisure and travel, recreation professionals thought that they would spend it on health care and investments. In any case, it is imperative that recreation professionals consider both economic levels and discretionary income of the baby boomer cohort, as leisure participation and program success today is largely based on the financial capabilities of the participant and the agency.

Together, these findings suggest what professionals know and don't know, helping to answer the question "Are you ready for boomers?" In the next section we discuss the values that boomers seek through leisure participation.

Boomer Leisure Values

Boomer leisure values were reflected in their responses to a series of statements in CBBQ 1 regarding the importance of their leisure participation. Each statement was related to either competitive, educational, physiological, social, relaxation, or aesthetic nonmoral leisure values. The results were analyzed by gender. These were some noteworthy findings:

1. Competitive values: Women (28 percent) considered participation in leisure for risk and adventure less important than did men (40 percent).

2. Educational values: Men were undecided about participating in leisure for purposes of creativity (35 percent), while women considered this important (44 percent).

3. Physiological values: Responses of both men and women indicated that they seek physical health, exercise, and relaxation (of mind, body, and spirit) through leisure experiences.

4. Social values: Both men and women (35 percent) indicated that they feel the social aspect is important during leisure.

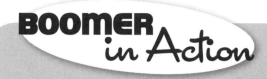

Cindy Heath

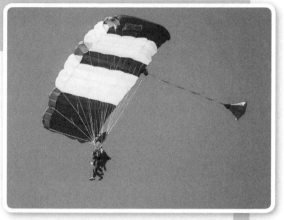

Turning 50 is certainly cause for celebration. At least it was for me. As the saying goes, "When opportunity knocks." And so it was, on a cloudless, sunny day in September, that I decided to jump out of a plane with the dual goal of supporting the Amani Children's Home in Tanzania and reflecting on a half-century of life experience. Granted, I never would have done this without a worthy cause. Nor would I have chosen to free-fall at 120 miles per hour from 10,000 feet toward a bumpy field in western Massachusetts without being securely attached to a charming and experienced jump instructor. Indeed, turning 50 has its advantages.

Along with the intense trepidation and heart-pounding fear I felt standing at the open door of the plane preparing to be launched into the sky, I allowed myself to experience just a little well-deserved pride. A healthy sense of adventure and seeking experiences that take us outside our comfort zone keep us energized and inspired. And if we can contribute to enriching the lives of children while we grow ourselves, well, that's just icing on the cake. So here's an open invitation to join me in next year's Jump For Amani—an experience you won't soon forget.

Profile and photo courtesy of Cindy Heath.

5. Relaxation values: Men (48 percent) and women (51 percent) both ranked relaxation values as important, and neither indicated that relaxation for the purpose of being away from family was important.

6. Aesthetic values: More than 50 percent of both male and female boomers indicated that they look to leisure for pleasure and for enjoyment of nature.

Again, the results emphasize in general what boomers are about. In the next section we discuss more particular leisure activity interests of boomers.

Leisure Activity Interests

In the questions about boomers and particular leisure activities, boomers were asked to identify the leisure activities that they currently participated in, and recreation professionals were asked what leisure activities they *thought* boomers participated in. Responses were classified by common leisure categories: art, crafts, dance, drama, music and rhythm, nature and outings, sports and games, educational activities, service activities, fitness, and others (those not represented by a category).

Table 2.1 reflects the top 10 leisure activities that boomers participated in at the time and the recreation professionals' perspective on the top 10 leisure activities that boomers participated in (ordered from highest to lowest).

Further, the top 10 leisure activities that boomers would like to participate in during retirement were identified; 60 percent of boomers felt that they would continue the same activities they were currently engaged in. Additional interests are shown below in ranking from popular preference to the least popular and examples are given for each category.

1. Sports and games: Boomers were interested in surfing, playing bridge, paragliding, learning to fly, rafting, running a marathon, tennis, swimming, and skydiving.
2. Travel: Questions did not address specifics on travel, although 32 percent of boomers indicated interest in pursuing travel or doing more traveling during their retirement.
3. Nature outings: Boomers identified boating (canoe, kayak), camping, fishing, hiking and backpacking, river running, bungee jumping, climbing, and hang gliding.

Table 2.1   Top 10 Leisure Activities Boomers Enjoy Now

Boomers' perspective	Recreation professionals' perspective
Reading	Travel
Walking	Fitness
Gardening	Walking
Travel	Golf
Hiking	Social activities
Bicycling	Taking university courses
Social activities	Reading
Movies	Investments and finance
Camping	Music
Sewing or music	Bicycling or gardening

4. Crafts: Boomers remained interested in crafts—cooking, craft activities in community classes, glass fusion.

5. Education: Responses indicated that boomers were interested in owning their own business, creative writing, learning a new language, or going back to school.

6. Music: While many desired to continue with current leisure interests in music, 5 percent of boomers expressed an interest in learning how to play an instrument during retirement.

Recreational professionals identified the top 10 leisure activities that they felt boomers would like to participate in during retirement. Seventy percent felt that boomers would continue the same activities that they were currently involved in; additional interests are shown below in ranking by popular preference and examples are given for each category—no additional notations were made to art, crafts, dance, or drama.

1. Sports and games: These included golf, walking, tennis, bowling, swimming, and bicycling or boating (canoe, kayak).

2. Travel: Though questions did not address specifics on travel, 23 percent of recreation professionals indicated that they felt boomers would pursue travel or engage in more travel during their retirement.

3. Nature outings and education: Nature activities included fishing, gardening, hiking, hunting, and camping. Leisure activities involving education included going back to school, finances, and reading.

4. Fitness and social: Only 8 percent of recreation professionals felt boomers would work out at the gym or spend time with family and friends.

5. Service and other: Involvement during retirement in politics, environmental issues, volunteering, or part-time work were service activities that recreation professionals (6 percent) felt boomers would participate in during retirement. Six percent also indicated that boomers would be interested in activities involving museums and parks, shopping, hobbies, and television.

In summary, boomers identified movies, camping, and sewing as among their top 10 current activities, whereas recreation professionals identified taking university courses and spending time on investments and finance. Boomers listed several activities that may be considered unusual and that recreation professionals did not list, such as riding ATVs, gambling, wine making, berry picking, bird watching, visiting hot springs, going to farmers' markets, and climbing. Clearly, boomers currently participated in more active leisure activities than recreation professionals believed they did; and recreation professionals appeared to view boomers as similar to the older senior population, taking classes and spending time on finances.

Regarding retirement, boomers stated that they would participate in crafts, while recreation professionals felt that boomers would volunteer or participate in fitness activities more. Also, boomers indicated that during retirement they would like to try surfing, paragliding, running a marathon, skydiving, river running, bungee jumping, hang gliding, owning a business, learning a new language, and learning how to play a musical instrument. Clearly the boomer expectations indicate a healthy, vibrant lifestyle.

As the results show, boomers plan to carry their willingness to learn new things, their desire for challenge, and their passion for education and culture with them into retirement. Evidence suggests that recreation professionals need to have an understanding that boomers' leisure activity interests are not the same as those of the traditional senior.

Boomers are active, dynamic, and highly educated. Their finances are sound, and they live life to its fullest. They plan to learn new things, seek challenges, and continue educational and cultural pursuits during retirement. Together, the results on nonmoral leisure values and leisure activity interests of boomers clearly provide a strong defense for the need to develop a different philosophical lens, a values-based lens, when we are providing leisure programs and services to the baby boomer cohort.

ARE YOU READY FOR BOOMERS?

We often focus on our participants as we prepare for leisure programming. We also need to focus on ourselves. Leisure programming starts with our agencies, our readiness as professionals to deliver. The second part of Cochran Baby Boomer Quiz 2 addresses the overall preparedness on the part of professionals and agencies in relation to their leisure programming, their facilities, and their services for baby boomers. This section included 10 questions. Frequencies were used for evaluation of responses. Results showed that 62 percent of recreation professionals have considered the boomer impact, with 91 percent agreeing that boomers will demand more than what our current senior centers and retirement communities are providing.

Three questions using a Likert scale (1 = low, 5 = high) prompted recreation professionals to rate themselves, their staff, and their agency on boomer knowledge, confidence, and preparedness for this new cohort. The questions and responses were as follows:

CBBQ 2, part 2, question 3: "Do you feel confident, with your knowledge about this generation, that you can provide adequate programs, services, and facilities?" Forty-one percent of the respondents rated themselves at level 3, representing an average score.

CBBQ 2, part 2, question 4: "Rate your staff on confidence about this generation and providing adequate programs, services, and facilities." Only 36 percent indicated a level 3 on the Likert scale for this question, and only 5 percent indicated a level 5, a high score.

CBBQ 2, part 2, question 5: "How do you rate your agency's preparedness for the growing aging population and leisure services?" Interestingly, 4 percent indicated a level 1 for their agency's preparedness while 40 percent indicated a level 3 for agency preparedness.

Together, these results do not reflect strong confidence about boomer knowledge on the part of recreation programmers or their staffs. As for agency preparedness, the results may suggest that recreation agencies are not fully ready for boomers. This adds fuel to the fire: We need to take a proactive philosophical approach to leisure programming for boomers—now!

In this chapter we have discussed how to identify nonmoral leisure values as reflected in our current literature, and how recreation professionals can assess their boomer population and also themselves as professionals. We have reviewed data supporting the development of a new assessment tool and the need for a philosophical approach to leisure programming via consideration of values. In the next chapter we discuss the use of values within marketing.

3

Marketing to Baby Boomers

You've begun to understand the massive potential of the baby boomer market. Baby boomer marketing strategist Jim Gilmartin pointed to the enormity of the boomer population when he wrote, "Baby Boomers are turning 50 at an astonishing rate of 1 every 10 seconds. That's more than 12,000 each day and over 4 million a year for each year of the next decade!" (Gilmartin, 2007, Home page). Apart from their sheer numbers, the boomers are also a generation of spenders that park, recreation, and leisure marketers must not ignore. Current statistics estimate their combined spending power at an overwhelming $1 trillion per year. Boomers also represent over 27 percent of the U.S. population and make up 46 million households.

This book deals throughout with how to create and enhance programs and leisure products to better meet the needs of the 76 million baby boomers, today and as they age. But, as you improve the way you program for boomers, you must also take a fresh look at the strategies you will use to promote or "sell" these programs to this important and powerful demographic.

In his bestselling book *The Art of the Deal,* baby boomer business tycoon Donald Trump (1989) says, "You can have the most wonderful product in the world, but if people don't know about it, it's not going to be worth much. You need to generate interest, and you need to create excitement" (p. 43). The same holds true for recreation programs and services. As you retool your recreation products to better meet, or even exceed, the needs of your baby boomer customers, you must also rethink the way you will promote these programs.

Keep in mind that according to baby boomer marketing expert Jim Gilmartin, "These baby boomers collectively make up the wealthiest, best educated, most sophisticated generation of consumers ever known. To win their business, you must create compelling communications, motivating messages and stellar customer service programs to better capture and keep current and potential customers" (Gilmartin, 2008, Home page).

IMPLEMENTING SUCCESSFUL MARKETING

By definition, marketing is everything you do to get and keep your customers. Marketing is much more than advertising, promotion, public relations, and the Internet (Rudick, 2000). It is not just about attracting customers and getting their money. Rather, successful marketing—especially as it relates to baby boomers—relies on the ultimate goal of developing long-term, even lifelong, customer relationships.

The Four P's of Marketing

The "Four P's of Marketing—Product, Price, Place, Promotion" have been part of the marketing vernacular for more than half a century (Borden, 1964). These four P's are known as the marketing mix and are a good place to begin your marketing planning process.

Today, however, there are many more concepts that make up the marketing mix, especially as it relates to service-based businesses such as recreation and leisure agencies. By adding four more P's—People, Planning, Perspective, and Philosophy—to the mix, you ensure a more comprehensive approach to your marketing communications strategies, especially as they relate to a population as powerful as boomer consumers (Rudick, 2007; see figure 3.1).

When you are evaluating marketing results—successes or failures—this expanded marketing mix enables you to explore much more than your promotional activities. In other words, if your programs aren't filling up the way you'd hoped, the problem may not rest in your promotions alone—brochure, Web site, or ads. The problem may lie in one of the other P's. These are some of the possibilities:

- Your *price* may be too high for retirees on a fixed income.
- Your *place* might be geographically inconvenient.
- It may be that your *product* itself needs to be retooled to meet changing boomer needs.
- Your *people* (staff or volunteers) may lack the motivation, enthusiasm, or training to effectively serve your boomer customers.
- Your communication *plan* or marketing strategy may be outdated or may require new, cutting-edge media to reach tech-smart boomers.
- You may need to gain clearer customer *perspective,* including a better understanding of your competition and the overall marketplace.
- You may even need to take a hard look at your agency's overall mission or *philosophy* to make sure it aligns with changing community needs

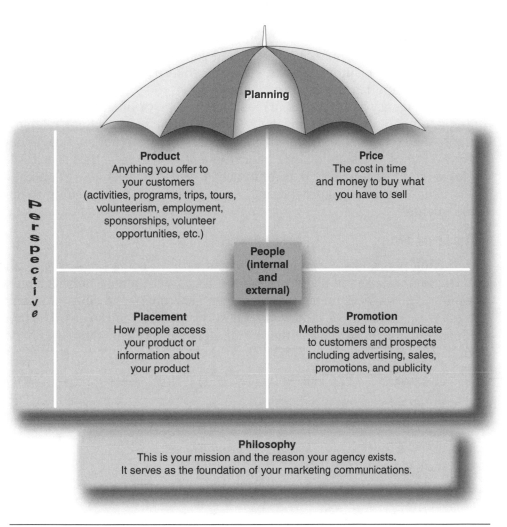

Figure 3.1 The eight P's of marketing: a holistic approach.

and populations. For example, your recreation agency may offer an extensive inventory of programs for children and youth but offer little for adults beyond the occasional athletic league. Now may be the perfect time to retool your mission statement, emphasizing *your philosophy of providing equal access to all citizens—including grown-ups!* You may even choose to enhance your mission statement and specifically address the growing needs of your growing boomer population.

A Marketing Blueprint

A marketing plan is like a blueprint for your organization's future, giving it structure and framework. Just like an architect's blueprint, the marketing plan provides a concrete picture of promotional strategies, goals, and outcomes. It answers the question "Where do we want to go for programming?"

This written plan is especially useful for multifaceted organizations, as it allows everyone—from front-line staff and volunteers to board members and administrators—to understand the steps you collectively need to take to build your most important asset, your customer base.

If your agency has a master plan, strategic plan, or other long-term planning document, take it off the shelf. If the plan includes sections related to marketing communications, public awareness, or customer service, review those sections. You should also explore these reports to see if they specifically address your organization's commitment to the baby boomer population. Whenever possible, your marketing plan should align with existing agency documents.

Types of Plans

Marketing plans, like customers and organizations, come in all shapes and sizes. Some marketing plans address the needs of an entire organization or "brand." Others focus on a specific program area, division, facility, or product segment (aquatics, trails, rentals, athletics, cultural arts, and so on). The most effective plans, however, are those that focus on a specific target audience such as

- children,
- preadolescents and teenagers,
- baby boomers,
- active seniors,
- frail seniors, or
- community partners or business sponsors.

Historically, park and recreation agencies have focused on the needs of children. However, boomers, by sheer numbers alone, deserve their own marketing strategy. They are not seniors and are certainly not youth. Yet as we discussed in chapter 2, few agencies have given them the attention they deserve, as a separate, unique, fun-loving, recreation-seeking demographic.

If you are truly committed to attracting and retaining a strong and loyal boomer customer base, then you must design a targeted marketing plan specific to this end. Boomers will not respond to a one-size-fits-all marketing strategy any more than teenagers respond to dull, outdated, "old-school" marketing. Boomers, as they have done throughout their whole lives, will choose to "do business" with organizations that understand who they are and what they want. Today's boomers are especially apt to respond to marketing messages that speak directly to them.

Your Marketing Plan Template

There are hundreds of books, seminars, computer programs, Web sites, and consultants that can help you develop a sophisticated marketing plan. But don't overcomplicate your marketing planning process. Much of your plan is intuitive, based on your experience as a recreation specialist or programmer. You just need to take the time to write it down. While you may need to gather some data or do a bit of research, developing even a rough plan will launch you in a more strategic and effective direction.

A marketing plan is a fluid and flexible document. When developing your boomer-based marketing strategy, it is especially critical to review and update every 6 to 12 months. This will allow you to incorporate new media and technologies as well as give you the flexibility to improve programs based on customer feedback. Further, as your boomer population ages and their physical and emotional needs shift, you'll need to retool programs and promotions.

Take the time to review and complete the very simple marketing plan template presented in figures 3.2 and 3.3. Even this one-page plan will help you develop a more thoughtful approach to attracting baby boomer customers to your programs. This template explores the following key marketing components:

1. Objective: What will you accomplish with this marketing plan? What are your goals?
2. Target audience: Who will you reach?
    a. End users: Who are the people you directly serve?
    b. Gatekeepers: Who influences your end users (for example, doctors influence their patients, clergy influence members of their congregations, realtors influence new homeowners)?
3. Budget: How much money and time will you invest in order to reach your marketing goal?
4. Message: What will you "say" (through words, pictures, images, symbols, themes, illustrations, and so on) to get the attention of and motivate prospects to take action?
5. Marketing media: Where will you put your message?
6. Time line: When will marketing activities take place?

YOUR MARKETING MESSAGE

As you read this book you are enhancing your understanding of what makes baby boomers tick. You've learned about their history, their hot buttons, and their perspectives. As you develop your marketing tools and create offers, it's critical to incorporate your new-found boomer insight into all of your marketing materials.

As a marketer, it's your job to translate your programs' features into valuable benefits for your prospects and customers. Baby boomers especially need to know what's in it for them in order to want to participate in your programs and activities.

FIGURE 3.2 MARKETING PLAN TEMPLATE

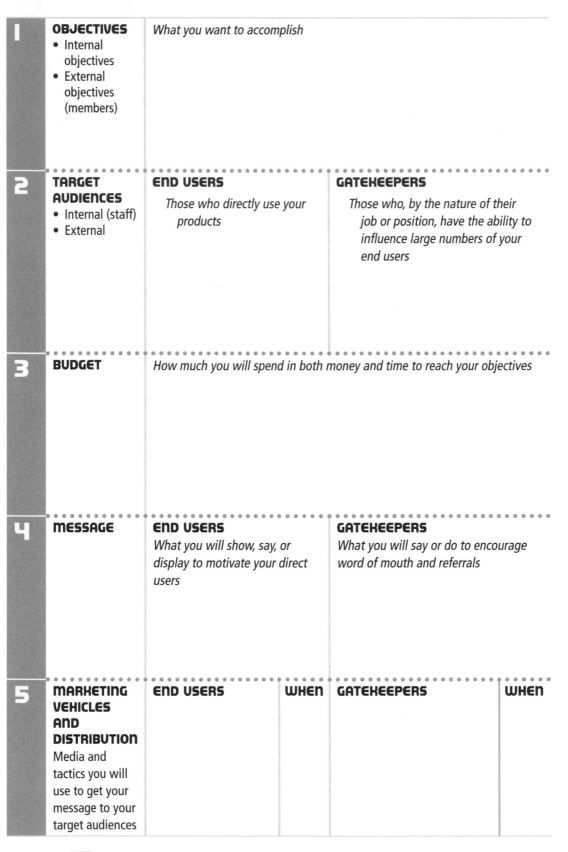

1 OBJECTIVES
- Internal objectives
- External objectives (members)

What you want to accomplish

2 TARGET AUDIENCES
- Internal (staff)
- External

END USERS

Those who directly use your products

GATEKEEPERS

Those who, by the nature of their job or position, have the ability to influence large numbers of your end users

3 BUDGET

How much you will spend in both money and time to reach your objectives

4 MESSAGE

END USERS
What you will show, say, or display to motivate your direct users

GATEKEEPERS
What you will say or do to encourage word of mouth and referrals

5 MARKETING VEHICLES AND DISTRIBUTION
Media and tactics you will use to get your message to your target audiences

END USERS	WHEN	GATEKEEPERS	WHEN

FIGURE 3.3 SAMPLE BABY BOOMER MARKETING PLAN

1	**OBJECTIVES** • External objectives (members)	*What you want to accomplish*	
		We want to increase the number of Baby Boomer Fitness Center memberships by 20% over the next 12 months.	

2	**TARGET AUDIENCES** • Internal (staff) • External	**END USERS**	**GATEKEEPERS**
		Those who directly use your products	*Those who, by the nature of their job or position have the ability to influence large numbers of your end users*
		We will focus on baby boomers who have recently been diagnosed with some type of cardiovascular disease or health concern (high blood pressure, cholesterol, obesity, and so on).	*Health care professionals* *Weight loss centers* *Pharmacies*

3	**BUDGET**	*How much you will spend in both money and time to reach your objectives*
		$2000 per quarter

4	**MESSAGE**	**END USERS**	**GATEKEEPERS**
		What you will show, say, or display to motivate your direct users	*What you will say or do to encourage word of mouth and referrals*
		We will position the fitness center as their lifesaver.	*Offer referral incentives* *Educate gatekeepers about the value of the fitness center for patients* *Give discounts to patients* *Discount memberships for health care professionals* *FREE passes for patients*

5	**MARKETING VEHICLES AND DISTRIBUTION** Media and tactics you will use to carry your message to your target audiences	**END USERS**	**WHEN**	**GATEKEEPERS**	**WHEN**
		• *Press releases to community papers, health and wellness publications* • *Special event in February to celebrate National Heart Month* • *Active living community advertising in monthly senior living magazines* • *Advertising in insurance publications* • *Exhibit at health and wellness expos*		• *Waiting room literature* • *Prescription pads* • *Calendars* • *Imprinted activity books* • *Sudoku, word jumbles for waiting room* • *Wall clocks for examination rooms* • *Sticky note pads* • *Imprinted bags with tear-off coupon to be used by pharmacies*	

Marketing Is Motivation

While boomers have distinct characteristics, the fact remains that all human beings share certain physiological and physical needs. In the mid-20th century, psychologists such as Abraham Maslow and Frederick Herzberg (Herzberg et al., 1959) began studying human behavior and motivation. In 1943 Maslow proposed a theory of motivation suggesting that behavior is determined by a wide variety of needs. According to Maslow, motivation starts when an individual experiences a need; the individual then formulates a goal, which, upon achievement, will satisfy the need. His hierarchy of needs (figure 3.4) illustrated how lower-level needs such as food, shelter, safety, and security must be satisfied, at least in part, before an individual begins to strive to satisfy needs at a higher level (Maslow, 1954).

It's no coincidence that marketing, as a discipline, emerged at the same time that Maslow and others were publishing their work. Marketing, after all, is about motivation, and smart marketers have learned to apply this psychology effectively to the business of selling products.

So while baby boomers tend to be more independent and self-reliant than other generations, they are not immune to outside motivators and influencers. However, boomers have always relied on past experiences and advice from peers when making consumer and life decisions, and they will continue to do so. They also will trust their own sets of beliefs and values to guide them through life.

Each and every day, messages enter our conscious and subconscious minds, swaying us to make choices and decisions. Ethical marketing does not manipulate, mislead, "bait and switch," or sabotage competitors. Rather,

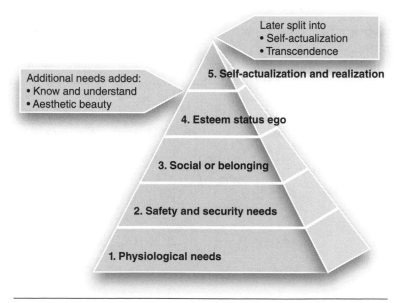

Figure 3.4 Maslow's hierarchy of needs.

fair marketing educates, informs, and guides customers to make choices that solve problems and enhance quality of life.

As a marketer, it's your job to translate your programs' features into valuable benefits and solutions for your prospects and customers. This is what will move them to act the way you want them to.

Moving Boomers to Action

By nature, boomers are inquisitive, self-focused, and demanding. As youth they fought against "the establishment," yet as adults they seemed to effortlessly and successfully become part of that very same corporate structure. Now, with more time on their hands, they may once again find themselves passionately searching for their social conscience.

So, what on earth will you say or do to motivate boomers to behave or act the way you want? How will you get them excited about what you have to offer? After all, they are very busy people. Their brains are already filled with millions of pieces of information, and every day they are bombarded with more and more input. What will you do to break through all this clutter?

As you create your marketing message or campaign, remember that your goal is to win your customers' attention and motivate them to take action by tapping into their needs—not yours. To successfully market and communicate to boomers, whether on the Web or face-to-face, it's critical to remember who they are and how they view the world.

Marketing materials that speak to these beliefs, values, and common experiences greatly increase the chances of breaking through communication clutter. You should consider the following list of baby boomer characteristics when developing marketing messages and choosing promotional tools:

- Grew up in a period of unprecedented prosperity
- Have unparalleled expectations of the future
- Believe in a lifestyle of free choice
- Are the most educated, influential, prosperous generation in U.S. history
- Desire to do things differently than their parents' generation did
- Are experimental and willing to try new things
- Will view retirement as an active period in their lives
- Believe in individualism and are rarely hesitant to voice their opinions
- Are patriotic and oriented toward social causes
- Have a work hard, play hard, spend hard mentality
- Have a sense of adventure and enjoy breaking the rules
- Want to remain in their own homes or own neighborhoods even as they age

- Seek entertaining education and lifelong learning
- Demand high-tech, state-of-the-art fitness centers
- Support walking trails, walkable communities, and on-site programming
- Will break through stereotypes of aging—aiming to look good and young forever
- Love style, pop culture, and rock 'n' roll
- Search for balance in holistic activities (mind, body, spirit)

The Boomer Brain

Boomers not only share certain beliefs, values, and experiences, but, says noted author and baby boomer expert David B. Wolfe, also have something else in common. "As we age," says Wolfe, "our brain physically changes" (p. 267). He stresses that people should take these changes into consideration when developing marketing messages and materials for older adults (Wolfe & Snyder, 2003).

Keep in mind that marketing, sales, and public relations are about getting information into people's brains that ultimately motivates them to buy or to take some other action. The older we become, says Wolfe, the more we are motivated by emotional rather than rational messages. Emotional triggers cause us to pay attention more often than information alone does. Emotional triggers in the brain activate memories, and the stronger the memory, the stronger the response. Marketing and sales must integrate both honesty and openness into marketing messages. These two attributes are necessary to build trust and are essential to optimal results in marketing and sales communications.

Understanding how a baby boomer's brain processes information is key to developing effective communications. Jim Gilmartin, owner of the nationally recognized baby boomer marketing firm Coming of Age, says, "If an ad, brochure, television or radio spot, Web site or sales presentation fails to connect with a baby boomer's idealized image of self, it is more likely to be ignored" (Gilmartin, 2007, Home page).

Specific changes in the baby boomer's aging brain create both opportunities and challenges for recreation marketers. These changes and their applications are illustrated in table 3.1.

A Boomer's Day—Breaking Through the Clutter

Whether you are a baby boomer or not, think about your typical day. From the time you wake up until the time you "hit the hay," your day is filled with obligation, responsibility, and commitments. Now think about a day in the life of the typical baby boomer. Although you would like to think that he or she is sitting around just waiting for your marketing message to come along, the truth is that today's baby boomer customer is very busy and occupied. While not common, it is actually possible for boomers to be caring

Table 3.1 The Boomer Brain

The Boomer Brain	Implications and Applications
Intuition trumps reason Boomers rely less on reason and trust their intuition.	• Identify and use images that promote strong positive emotional responses. • Build relationships with your customers by recognizing their feelings, concerns, and successes. • Show that you care before talking about product features or information about your agency.
You really never get a second chance to make a first impression Initial reactions (which are always emotionally based) are more enduring and therefore more difficult to reverse than for younger adults.	• Don't use images that can stimulate negative first impressions. • Don't use images that conflict with baby boomers' idealized image of self, especially with respect to autonomy and sense of personal validity. • Don't call boomers "seniors" or "old." • Do an on-site analysis of facilities to insure that they feel friendly, warm, and comfortable. • Don't display posters of people who look like traditional "seniors." • Boomers see themselves as 10 to 15 years younger than they are.
Hook 'em, reel 'em in After interest is piqued, baby boomers will want and seek more information than younger consumers.	• Once boomers are *emotionally* hooked, they need *rational* information to reinforce their buying decision. • Continue to weave and balance emotional and objective information throughout the buying process. Don't over-inform. • Offer options and resources that inquisitive boomers can go to for additional information.
Slow it down Rational processing of objective information decreases in speed with aging.	• Deliver objective information (e.g., product benefits, registration details, program features, rules, policies, technical information) at a slow to moderate pace. • Offer information in both written and verbal formats. • Use complete sentences.
No puffery, please Boomers are more resistant to absolute propositions than others.	• Present information about your organization, programs, and agency in a factual and objective manner. • Don't use hyperbole, puffery, or exaggeration. • Be prepared to prove claims and offer sources when sharing statistical information. • Use testimonials from real people who represent the idealized self-image.
Metaphors mean more Boomers are more sensitive to metaphorical meanings, nuances, and subtleties.	• Use humor, case histories, and double entendre. • Never insult their intelligence. • Use visuals (e.g., illustrations, graphics, and symbols) to create metaphorical meaning.

(continued)

Table 3.1 *(continued)*

The Boomer Brain	Implications and Applications
Tell me a story Boomers are more receptive to narrative-styled presentations of information, less responsive to information presented in expository style.	• Make greater use of storytelling techniques to get information across. Stories generally arouse emotions more quickly than straightforward propositions about a product's features. Think Hallmark Cards—they surpass most in using stories to present products. • Don't be emotionally neutral; spark a reaction. • Storytelling has become an important part of market strategy. • Whoever tells the best story and tells it best will most likely win.
Whole-person promotion Boomers' perceptions are more holistic.	• Project an interest in the "whole" person, not just the part of the person that needs parks, recreation, and leisure services. • Help people to find a solution or even do business with your competitor if you can't meet their needs. • Avoid depicting baby boomers as flat, single-dimensional caricatures (e.g., simply showing consumers using or talking about the product without reference to a larger context).

Adapted, by permission, from J. Gilmartin, 2002, "Eight progressive changes in how older minds process information." [Online]. Available: http://www.comingofage.com/Articles/articledocs/To_Increase_Sales-Tell_A_Story.pdf [December 23, 2008]. Previously adapted from several unpublished papers by David B. Wolfe.

for four generations of dependents—children, grandchildren, parents, and grandparents—all at the same time. More likely, however, boomers at some point in their lives will feel squeezed between two generations, juggling the needs of elderly parents as well as those of their own children.

So how do you get attention from those unaware baby boomer prospects? The key, according to behavioral scientists such as Abraham Maslow, B.F. Skinner, and Frederick Herzberg, is to tap into physical and emotional motivators.

Boomer customers, like all customers, want to feel excited, hopeful, exhilarated, and enthused. They participate in recreation programs to maintain health, improve their lives, or feel satisfaction—physically, mentally, and spiritually. Professional copywriting expert Edward O'Keefe says, "Let your customers *feel* danger. Fear. Heat. Sex. Hunger. Pain. Desire. Life. Death. Stoke them up, and then tell them how to get what they want. Fulfill that desire. Quench that thirst. Eliminate that pain. Easy. Fast. Free." O'Keefe stresses that advertising is about emotions: "You need to make your customers squirm, or wince, or laugh, or cry. From bad breath to a full-blown heart attack, advertisers use fear to motivate because it works" (O'Keefe, 2007, "34 Ways to Make Your Advertising More Effective" subheader).

So, breaking through the clutter may be as simple as reminding or educating prospects about emotional issues. Once they are emotionally engaged, it's your job to position your programs as the solution.

> Then you better start swimmin'
> Or you'll sink like a stone
> For the times they are a-changin'.
>
> —Bob Dylan, 1964
> "The Times They Are A-Changin'"

THE STEPS TO THE BUY

Gaining attention from customers is one thing. But getting them to actually register or to "buy" your program or product is another. Your own experience, apart from when you are in a supermarket checkout line, tells you that most purchases are not purely impulsive or spontaneous. Most of the time, we begin the buying process long before any money changes hands.

As consumers, we may research options, think things through, look for the best deal, and still procrastinate or stall. Baby boomers are no exception. While they may have decades of consumer experience, they still make buying decisions in phases or steps. Therefore, it's unlikely that a single marketing piece will generate results—especially when you are trying to attract new customers. In a 2006 study conducted by the public relations firm Fleishman-Hilliard, the "majority of boomers (76%) indicate[d] that they prefer[red] to get information about products and services from multiple sources" (FH Boom, 2006, "Point of View" subheader). To make almost any buying decision, consumers must go through at least six steps before they reach "The Buy."

For example, we believe (or are told) that we have a *problem* or are reminded we have a *need* (step 1). Eventually we have a *desire* to fix this problem or fill the need (step 2). Then, maybe we do some research to *gather options* (step 3) and *find the best solution* (step 4). If the *cost* makes sense (step 5) and the timing is right (step 6), then and only then do we *make a purchase* (final step). As illustrated in figure 3.5, the steps to the buy are a consumer's journey from problem to solution, desire to fulfillment, frustration to relief.

Now think of a typical baby boomer customer. Imagine the steps he or she will go through to get to your point of purchase or participation. Figure 3.6 further illustrates the steps to the buy for one hypothetical baby boomer customer. Notice the subtle transitions that move the customer from one step to the other, ultimately leading to a recreation decision.

Sometimes we complete all of the steps to the buy in a flash. Other times, we may take weeks, months, or years to complete the "transaction." Frequently we begin the process but fall off the buying ladder along the way.

As a marketer, it's your job to help your customers navigate the steps as easily as possible and help those who've lost their way. In many cases, the

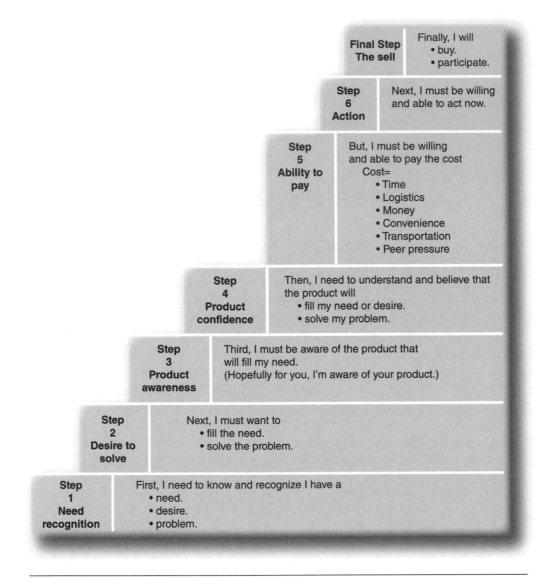

Figure 3.5 The steps to the buy.

key to new customer development is dependent upon your ability to nudge prospects to the first step on the buying ladder.

First Steps—Cause and Effect

First buying steps are often in response to a problem or a life-changing or milestone event. For today's baby boomer, these events aren't based so much on age as on their stage in life. Remember, too, that one person's cause for celebration might be another's crisis. Retirement, for example, causes joy and elation for some and feelings of loss, loneliness, or even grief in others.

Who: Male Baby Boomer   **What :** Fitness Center Membership

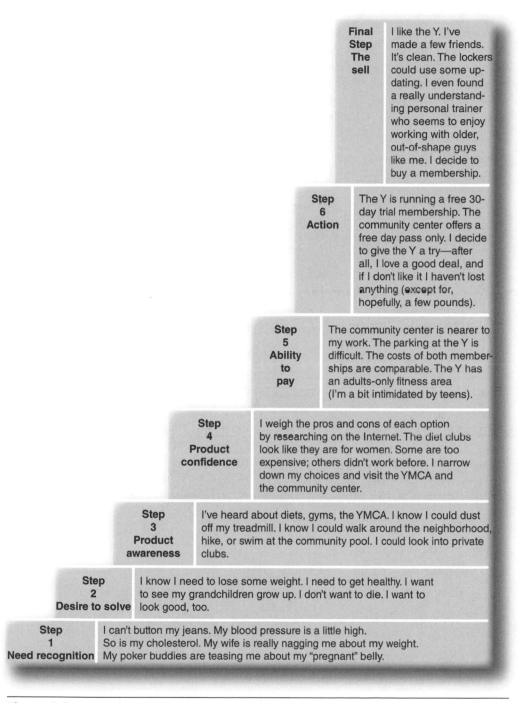

Final Step The sell

I like the Y. I've made a few friends. It's clean. The lockers could use some updating. I even found a really understanding personal trainer who seems to enjoy working with older, out-of-shape guys like me. I decide to buy a membership.

Step 6 Action

The Y is running a free 30-day trial membership. The community center offers a free day pass only. I decide to give the Y a try—after all, I love a good deal, and if I don't like it I haven't lost anything (except for, hopefully, a few pounds).

Step 5 Ability to pay

The community center is nearer to my work. The parking at the Y is difficult. The costs of both memberships are comparable. The Y has an adults-only fitness area (I'm a bit intimidated by teens).

Step 4 Product confidence

I weigh the pros and cons of each option by researching on the Internet. The diet clubs look like they are for women. Some are too expensive; others didn't work before. I narrow down my choices and visit the YMCA and the community center.

Step 3 Product awareness

I've heard about diets, gyms, the YMCA. I know I could dust off my treadmill. I know I could walk around the neighborhood, hike, or swim at the community pool. I could look into private clubs.

Step 2 Desire to solve

I know I need to lose some weight. I need to get healthy. I want to see my grandchildren grow up. I don't want to die. I want to look good, too.

Step 1 Need recognition

I can't button my jeans. My blood pressure is a little high. So is my cholesterol. My wife is really nagging me about my weight. My poker buddies are teasing me about my "pregnant" belly.

Figure 3.6   Example: Boomers step to the buy.

Table 3.2　Common Issues and Life Cycle Events

Problem	Life change	Milestone event
• My jeans are too tight • My school-age kids are driving me crazy. • My arthritis is really getting in the way of my tennis game. • My vision is deteriorating, making it hard to drive at night. • I live on a fixed income.	• Our kids are all grown and gone. • My husband's new job requires that he travel 50% of the time. • My single daughter has moved back into the house with her small children. • I have retired. • My 85-year-old mother has dementia and is coming to live with us.	• I have gotten remarried. • I have become a grandparent. • My last child graduated from university. • My parents are celebrating their 60th anniversary. • My granddaughter is getting married.

Table 3.2 offers examples of common issues and life cycle events that may propel baby boomers onto the first step of the buying ladder.

Call Them to Action Every Step of the Way

Think of your marketing as an invitation to get involved, do something, make a move. As you've learned, awareness is a step, not the end result of your marketing. Each and every message, promotion, ad, Web site, or press release should be written, designed, or formatted in such a way that your prospects feel compelled to do something. Don't make your prospects guess what you want them to do. Make it easy and convenient for them to respond to your message and continue up the steps to the buy. Often you'll want to motivate your baby boomer prospect to take one or more of the following specific steps in the ultimate journey toward a purchasing decision:

- Accept your call
- Attend a meeting
- Become a "friend" or virtual "friend"
- Complete a registration form or some other type of paperwork
- Send an e-mail
- Fill out a survey
- Give a referral
- Join an online network
- Log on to your Web site
- Make a call to someone else
- Post a comment on your blog

- Provide contact information for future marketing (a cell phone number for text messaging, e-mail address for e-mail promotions, street address for catalogs)
- Return forms via mail or e-mail
- Return your call
- Share information with someone else
- Sign up or register for a program, activity, or event
- Subscribe to a newsletter or blog feed
- Visit your facility or place of business
- Visit your trade show booth

No matter what your call to action, make it clear. Today's baby boomer customers are too busy to guess about or search for what you want them to do. Your "call to action" should lead your prospects to the next steps they need to take to improve their life.

CHOOSING MARKETING MEDIA

In the previous section you learned that marketing results depend upon how well your message resonates with baby boomer prospects to evoke emotion. But, once you have created a compelling message, theme, or concept, you must choose the best media to carry that message to your boomer prospects.

Never before have we seen so many new media choices emerge so quickly. No matter the terminology, the media mix is an ever-changing part of today's marketing landscape. Your activity guide, brochure, or catalog of classes is just one of hundreds of media options. Your Web site is another. Flyers may be a third media tool. But there are literally hundreds more avenues you can take to get your message in front of your customers.

Generation-by-Generation Comparison

All of the generations alive today grew up in very different media cultures. Most preboomers born before 1945 grew up listening to radio. Television was a luxury in the 1940s, and programming was limited to a few hours a day. By 1952 (as the firstborn baby boomers were entering grade school), television was beginning its golden age. As the boomers grew, so did their media options. They saw their world go from black and white to color and then to MTV. Today, of course, baby boomers have hundreds (maybe thousands) of media channels on television, on radio, on the Internet, via satellite, and on cell and video phones. Since the beginning of the new millennium we have moved from the information age into the participation age. Marketing is no longer mired in one-way messages but is rather a multifaceted, globally charged, completely interactive conversation. Today's consumers resist

Table 3.3 Boomer Modes of Media

To reach boomers (born 1946 to 1964)	**The majority of boomers (76%) indicate that they prefer to get information about products and services from multiple sources.**
	Combine traditional media with limited interactive media.

	• Newspapers
	• Radio
	  ◦ Classic rock
	  ◦ Talk, news, public radio
	• Magazines (such as *More* and *AARP: The Magazine*)
	• Direct mail
	• Newsletters
	• Billboards
	• E-mail
	• Banner ads
	• Cinema advertising
	• Television—one-third of boomers say television advertisements are the best way to reach them about new products and services

	The Internet is an equally powerful medium.
	Word of mouth and the ability to sample or test products firsthand have a strong impact on purchase decisions.

messages that are pushed at them. Instead they seek out and pull information toward them. To succeed in this digital age, you must go where they go—literally and figuratively, actually and virtually—in order to tell your story and connect to their emotions and needs. Table 3.3 offers a sample of media options best suited for reaching boomers.

Customers in Control

Ultimately, your customers and prospects determine which media you should use to deliver your message. Take the time to talk to or survey customers to find out the answers to these critical marketing questions:

- Where does your target audience get its information (radio, TV, specific newspapers, Web sites, friends, clergy, neighbors, health care professionals, business associates, and so on)?
- Where does your target audience "hang out"? Where do they go for entertainment and to socialize?
- What types of radio or television programs or what specific stations or channels do they listen to or watch?

- How do they make buying decisions about your particular product or service?

Other factors that will influence your media choices include the following:

- Your monetary budget
- Your time line
- Your "inventory," availability, or manpower
  - Be careful not to attract more customers than you and your team can feasibly handle (Waiting lists are NOT a marketing success!).
  - Baby boomers do not like being told no or that a class or event is full or sold out.
  - Boomers can be impatient and will not want to stand in line to register for a program.

The key to your marketing mix is to choose vehicles within your time and money budget that will work the best to reach your target audience.

Four Media Categories

While media can be categorized in many different ways, one of the most functional ways is to group them based on their reach or "intimacy." In order from narrow (most intimate) to wide (least intimate), these are the categories:

1. Sales communication
2. Promotions
3. Public relations
4. Mass media advertising

Some media may fall into more than one category. For instance, your Web site has the potential to reach mass, even global, audiences; but it also can include promotional tools such as contests, giveaways, or information about special events. You set up a promotional booth at your summer concerts. At the booth, of course, you engage visitors in one-on-one conversations that are part of the sales communication category. The categories themselves are not nearly as important as your willingness to explore and experiment with a variety of marketing strategies.

But remember, without the right message, nothing will work to move boomers to action! And even if your message is right on target, if your boomer prospects never see it, then your efforts will fail.

Sales Communication and Word-of-Mouth Marketing

Some marketing methods deliver one message at a time with little or no wasted exposure. Baby boomers are especially affected by the advice of those they trust and respect. Marketing lasers are those strategies that are delivered with pinpoint accuracy—usually face-to-face or person to person.

While most public recreation agencies don't have traditional sales departments, their counterparts in the travel and tourism profession often rely on sophisticated, well-trained salespeople to address customer needs and develop ongoing two-way relationships with prospects and clients. Whether through a formal or an informal sales system, every business or organization must engage in the sales process to communicate with prospects and customers.

Table 3.4 offers an overview of the most targeted media. The tactics listed, sometimes referred to as marketing lasers, include the most traditional tactics

Table 3.4　Sales Process

Characteristics	• Have pinpoint accuracy • Involve little or no monetary investment • Involve high time investment • Allow for immediate response • Enable two-way communication
Best for:	• Building relationships with end users and gatekeepers • Qualifying prospects • Gathering information • Using with people who have less money, lots of time • Finalizing details • Inexpensive ongoing communication (Note that some training is required to increase effectiveness.)
Marketing laser beams	• Personal visits • Interior point-of-purchase signage and displays • Exterior storefront signage • Canvassing and cold calls • Sales calls • Physical visits to the customer's home or business • Telemarketing • Personal letters and notes • Collateral packages (brochures, business cards, invoices, and so on) • Networking • Instant messaging • Text messaging • Personal Web sites (e.g., MySpace.com) • Blogs • Specialty advertising, gifts, and promotional items: 　○ Delivered by mail to individuals 　○ Delivered by customer pickup 　○ Delivered as part of a package

(door-to-door sales) and new and emerging media methods (text messaging, online social networks, and so on).

A Word About Word of Mouth

It seems that not a day goes by without our hearing about some new-fangled communication gizmo or gadget. Never before have we seen so many technological advances in the way we exchange information. With all these new technologies come new opportunities and new challenges. Clutter continues to rise, making it harder and harder for your message to break through.

Although new, high-tech marketing options seem to be entering the marketplace at laser-light speed, one thing remains constant. Word of mouth remains the most powerful and influential form of marketing. However, as interactive Web 2.0 technology becomes more and more mainstream, it will be necessary to use both organic (face-to-face, nonelectronic, traditional) word-of-mouth tactics and amplified (blogs, podcasts, social networking sites, and so on) word-of-mouth tools.

Boomers not only rely on advice and recommendations from others when making purchasing decisions; they also enjoy sharing their opinions with others. According to a recent study conducted by Weber Shandwick (Gaines-Ross, 2007), a global public relations firm, "A majority of baby boomers get asked for recommendations on products and services about 90 times every year. Nearly all (89%) of those who were asked for advice gave it to their friends, or fellow boomers. And nearly all boomers (93%) say that they consider their friends (also boomers) to be trusted sources of information." Explains Weber Shandwick Chief Reputation Strategist Dr. Leslie Gaines-Ross, "When it comes to word-of-mouth recommendations, boomers have both unrivaled influence and rich networks of peer advisors. As with most word-of-mouth, 84% of boomer recommendations are made face-to-face and 82% by phone, while only 45% are made online" (Gaines-Ross, 2007, report subheader).

While boomers may prefer organic word of mouth when making purchasing decisions, they frequently and increasingly use the Internet to research and compare products or services. The key to creating word of mouth in the digital age is to provide enough information online to fuel an offline word-of-mouth campaign.

PROMOTIONAL MARKETING TOOLS

When chosen correctly, most promotional tools have the power to motivate baby boomer customers to action. Promotional tools are precise and very effective when you are attempting to reach specific targets with common needs and values. Baby boomers respond well to promotional tools for many reasons.

First, these tools often allow for two-way conversation (trade shows; presentations; direct response and sampling, which allow respondents to offer an immediate opinion). Second, promotions can be customized and personal, appealing to the boomers' sense of individualism and style. Third, promotions, by definition, may involve discounts, price consideration, or premiums, which appeal to the boomers' sense of esteem and self-worth. The characteristics and uses of promotional media are illustrated in table 3.5 along with a list of common promotional options.

Table 3.5 Promotional Media

Characteristics of promotion	• Is very accurate • Enables direct response • Allows easy measurement of effectiveness • Varies in time and cost commitment • Is three dimensional • Is multisensory • Is permanent
Best for:	• Business-to-business marketers • Opening doors with gatekeepers and end users • Continuity and theme development • Establishing position and competitive edge • Follow-up to initial contact • Targeting marketing specialists

Examples	• Direct mail
	• Promotional products:
	  ◦ Delivered by mail
	  ◦ Delivered door to door
	  ◦ Delivered by local services, parcel services, and so on
	• Trade publications
	• Trade directories and newsletters
	• Self-published newsletters
	• Seminars
	• Speaking engagements
	• Demonstrations
	• Trade shows
	• Exhibits
	• Flea markets
	• Sampling
	• Bulletin boards at places where customers live, work, and play
	• Online bulletin boards
	• Yellow pages
	• Point of purchase
	• Electronic messaging (e.g., e-mail, IM, or text message), outgoing voicemail message, messages while on hold (e.g., instead of music)

Publicity and Public Relations

Publicity refers to free (vs. purchased) space and time given to businesses or organizations in exchange for information, education, and news. Public relations also refers to the broader marketing function of creating and developing your image or brand in the eyes of your various publics, such as baby boomers. It refers to your overall brand identity, including your public's perception of your organization. Your public image can vary from group to group. Mothers may feel that your organization and programs are extremely valuable while the empty-nest baby boomer may perceive your agency to be of little or no personal value. Historically, your agency may be oriented toward youth, leading boomers to feel disconnected with it.

Always remember that your public's perception is their reality. So, if you do augment your program inventory and begin offering programs for today's baby boomers, you will need to engage in a targeted public relations campaign to reeducate and correct years of preconceived notions or misperceptions. Table 3.6 presents a variety of publicity tools beyond the traditional press release, as well as the characteristics of public relations media.

Table 3.6   Publicity and Public Relations Media

Characteristics	• Are free • Vary in accuracy • Are difficult to control • Require time commitment (for writing news releases) • Involve monetary commitment if firm is hired to generate publicity • Come with no guarantees
Best for:	• Establishing credibility • Increasing awareness • Announcing a unique service or product • Supporting other marketing vehicles • Establishing position and competitive edge • Use by those with writing skills or the budget to employ a skilled publicist

Examples	• News releases to:
	  • Print media
	  • Broadcast media
	• Speaking to nonprofit groups
	• Giving interviews on radio and television programs
	• Making charitable contributions
	• Sponsoring teams and nonprofit special events
	• Getting actively involved with community and political organizations
	• Writing, commenting on, and contributing to Web logs (i.e., blogs)

Mass Media Marketing

Mass media marketing tools can hit a broad target with a lesser degree of accuracy. They tend to be more costly and are best used by marketers who are trying to reach large generic audiences. Fortunately, today there are many more mass media options for targeting baby boomers than ever before (see table 3.7).

It seems that currently all marketers, from cable television programmers to magazine publishers, are reinventing themselves to appeal to the baby boomer market with its multimillions in spending ability.

Table 3.7   Mass Media Marketing

Characteristics	• Are inaccurate (high degree of wasted exposure)
	• Reach the masses
	• Allow quick response
	• May entail high expense per ad but relatively low cost per thousand
	• For electronic media, effectiveness difficult to measure
	• For print media, effectiveness easy to measure via coupons
	• Require frequency
	• Must get through lots of clutter
	• Can be multisensory
Best for:	• Consumer marketers with wide target
	• Those with no time but lots of money to invest
	• Creating mass awareness with less need for action
Examples	• Newspapers
	• Network television
	• Cable television
	• Radio
	• Magazines
	• Outdoor and transportation
	• Widely distributed direct mail
	• Web site banner ads
	• Spam (mass e-mail marketing)

RETAINING CUSTOMERS

Your overall marketing effectiveness is not only about attracting new prospects. Baby boomers, especially, expect to be treated with care, respect, and appreciation throughout the entire transaction—before, during, and after the sale.

Customer development is a cyclical process. As you develop your marketing plan, craft your message and carefully choose media. You must also assess your ability to deliver—even overdeliver—on your promises.

While good, creative, well-placed marketing materials are great, they are a waste of money and time if front-line staff aren't equipped to handle incoming calls and customer questions. Further, if your actual programs and activities don't live up to your promotional promises, your baby boomer customers won't want to return. Worse than that, unhappy customers—especially opinionated boomers—will tell their friends, neighbors, and colleagues, creating a word-of-mouth disaster. Even with the flashiest Web site, the coolest blog, and the slickest brochure, nothing makes up for bad word of mouth. What's the moral? Strive for happy customers—every day, every session, every time.

You, as well as each and every member of your staff, need to understand and believe in the benefits of your products and programs. No matter what your job description, you are part of the marketing mix. Figure 3.7 illustrates the customer development process. Train staff to understand and be able to identify their impact on customers—even if they work behind the scenes. In other words, you've got to hook 'em, reel 'em in, and keep 'em coming back for more.

Baby boomers, known for their egocentric personalities, can be high-maintenance customers. They love customization and individual attention. To win their loyalty, you and your entire staff must fine-tune customer service skills. As customers, boomers want to do business with those who will listen

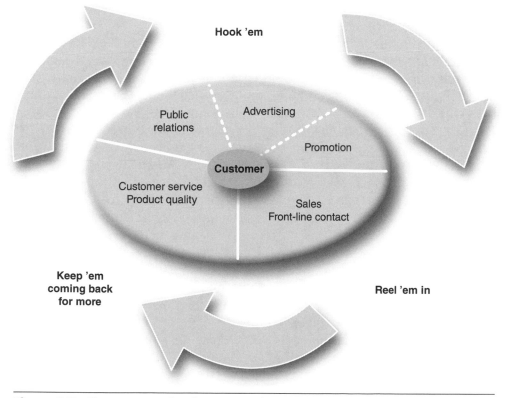

Figure 3.7 The customer development cycle.

and will value their opinion. They love being "right," which means that when boomers bring forward a complaint or suggestion, they want to hear that their opinion is valid. Boomers also are inquisitive, so when they ask a question about policies or procedures, be prepared to explain the reason behind the rules. There's no better way to aggravate a boomer than to respond with a curt "Because that's our policy" or "It's not my department."

Further, boomers, who have a natural tendency to question authority, will not appreciate being told "You can't fight city hall." After all, in their youth, boomers were notorious for questioning authority and challenging the "establishment." They marched for civil rights, protested against the Vietnam War, and forced corporations to become more environmentally responsible.

This means going beyond "please" and "thank you" when it comes to customer service. However, boomers are also more loyal than younger generations. So, those businesses, organizations, and people that treat boomers right will be amply rewarded with long-term, dedicated customers. It's extremely important to follow up with baby boomer customers. Good follow-up shows attention to detail and demonstrates your commitment to their needs.

Marketing is a process. It is about changing minds, behaviors, and attitudes. As you look back at your agency's marketing history, you may see that you have tried many different marketing ideas to bring in new customers. Some of them worked. Others did not. Marketing is also about patience, perseverance, and consistency. Strategies that failed in the past might deserve another look. Perhaps your ideas were ahead of their time.

Marketing is part science, part art, part intuition, and part luck. Remember the words of baby boomer icon Bob Dylan, "The times they are a-changin'." (When it comes to boomers, so are their minds, bodies, lifestyles, and families.) Timing *is* everything. What one person needs today may be obsolete next week. Your next customer may be shopping around or procrastinating. Potential customers may be very busy, or distracted, or broke, or tired. They may be on vacation. They may have just forgotten or misplaced your information. They may not be ready, or maybe they're not comfortable trusting you yet. It may take a few exposures to your message to get the action you want. Don't give up without giving your vehicle a fair chance to work.

As boomers age, they will experience many changes and milestones in their lives. Each of these milestones may prompt them to search for new recreation-based programs, products, and services. It is unlikely that one technique alone will get your customers to beat a path to your door. Memorability depends on the frequency and permanence of your message. Combine sales, marketing, promotion, and public relations to establish a strong position and build your boomer base.

Finally, remember that boomers will choose to do business with organizations that value and appreciate them before, during, and after the sale. Train staff to listen to and address their needs as the holistic and powerful consumers that they are.

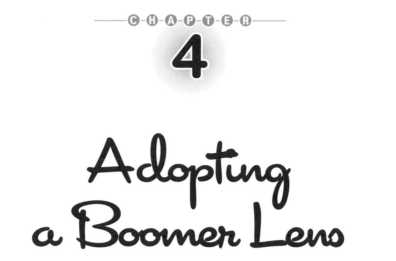

Adopting a Boomer Lens

The future of leisure programming and marketing focuses on a population that will be more active than recreation professionals are currently ready for. It is important for recreation professionals to rethink their method of identifying, developing, implementing, and recruiting the boomer generation to their leisure programs. We also need to rethink how we instruct our future recreation professionals in the classroom. While boomers plan to carry into retirement their willingness to learn new things, their desire for challenge, and their passion for education and culture, research indicates that recreation professionals need to examine different avenues for programming that will be more specific to the values of boomers and beyond those of today's traditional seniors.

By neglecting the very values of the cohorts they aim to serve, programmers will miss the mark as to providing key leisure opportunities that their participants desire and deserve. By examining the boomer generation's values and beliefs relative to leisure pursuits, we will have a more reflective and philosophical stance from which to develop appropriate and meaningful leisure programming for this cohort. Thus it is important for us to adopt a philosophical lens—a boomer lens—when designing and implementing leisure programs. We must consider a values-based programming philosophy that produces identifiable outcomes as discussed in chapter 2.

Adopting a "boomer lens" will allow you to understand who boomers are, what boomers are doing, and where boomers are going, as well as when and how they will do what they do. Do you have a funky pair of sunglasses? Dig them out, put them on, and get ready to see through the lens of a boomer! We have already discussed what drives boomers, as well as marketing techniques for attracting boomers and getting them in your door. Figure 4.1 revisits the

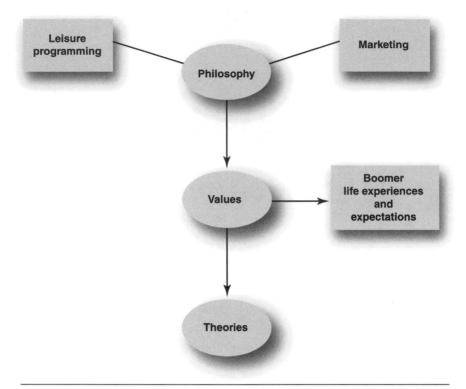

Figure 4.1 The relationship of the elements which created a boomer lens.

relationship of boomers' values to the need for a programming philosophy aimed at this approach.

The use of a "boomer lens" will allow you to

- understand and create programs and marketing plans that are responsive to an unusual aging society,
- develop an awareness of external opportunities and challenges that will foster innovation and a positive response to serving a new clientele of participants, and
- consider the specific value structures of a new cohort.

Using a boomer lens, this chapter presents guidelines that will help you as a recreation professional position your organization to provide successful boomer programming. These guidelines involve three main steps:

1. Study the boomer picture.
2. Assess your agency's preparedness.
3. Strategize for boomer programming, marketing, and implementation.

GUIDELINES FOR BABY BOOMER LEISURE PROGRAMMING

With bodies aging but spirits still strong, baby boomers, as we emphasize throughout this book, are changing the face of recreation and leisure in many ways. As baby boomers march toward retirement, keep in mind that at every life stage they have rewritten the rules. They are going to do it again. The boomer generation is going to demand more than what our current senior centers and leisure programs are providing. Boomers will not be satisfied with a "regularly scheduled program" as often found in today's senior centers. Therefore, the approach to leisure programming and use of leisure facilities will have to break from the traditional norms to meet the demands of the baby boomer generation. Recreation professionals will be obligated to develop a large range and scope of adult-focused recreational activities, targeted at a program philosophy that entails the psychological, educational, physiological, social, and demographic interests of this new cohort.

Given the uniqueness of the boomer cohort and the future demand for leisure programs and services, this section presents important guidelines aimed at helping recreation professionals and their departments provide leisure programs and leisure services for the baby boomer cohort. The term *guidelines* as used in recreation can mean (a) a set of recommended actions to follow in implementing current policies, enabling agencies to enforce those policies; (b) various guiding principles for making recreation department

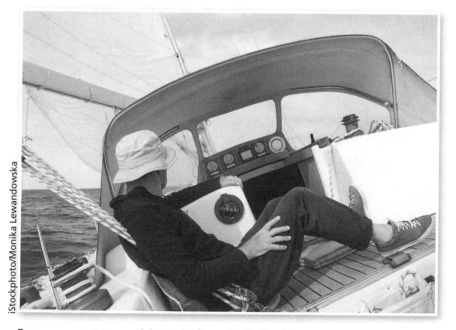

iStockphoto/Monika Lewandowska

Boomers want to participate in fun, physical, adventurous activities that will take them out of their comfort zone and challenge them.

programs safe and enjoyable for all participants; or (c) an organizational measurement designed to increase the quality of programs or facilities. With this in mind, in the following pages we discuss guiding principles based on a clearer philosophical lens derived from the Cochran Baby Boomer Quizzes 1 and 2 (see appendix).

These guiding principles provide recommended actions that we can take in order to meet the challenges associated with the baby boomer cohort. But, although adhering to only traditional theories or past approaches is not recommended, recreation professionals should not forget that the foundation of basic leisure programming concepts can be useful if modified. Therefore, some of the principles presented within this chapter are adapted for the boomer cohort from those that have traditionally appeared in textbooks, recreation program manuals, or similar sources, and also have been developed based on extensive amounts of combined hands-on leisure programming experience on the part of the authors.

Study the Boomer Picture

The baby boomer cohort, those born between 1946 and 1964, has dominated American culture for the past five decades. Every time boomers have taken a step, the spotlight of the media has swiveled to illuminate them. The massive numbers of their generation have amplified and intensified the importance of their experiences at each new moment in their lives. When boomers reach any stage of life, the issues that concern them, whether financial, interpersonal, or even hormonal, have become the dominant social, political, and marketplace themes of the time. Boomers do not just occupy existing life stages or consumer trends—they redefine them.

> **How can you consider flower power outdated? The essence of my lyrics is the desire for peace and harmony. That's all anyone has ever wanted. How could it become outdated?**
> —*Robert Plant*

One of the most important things known about boomers is that they are rule breakers. Individuality over conformity is a consistent pattern among boomers. They have always experienced life differently from the cohorts before them or from those who are following today. Their vast numbers have created fierce competition for everything they have wanted throughout their lives: for school space as children, for team and club memberships as teenagers, for university entrance, for homes and good careers as young adults. Boomers have transformed the food, automobile, and fashion industries; education; the workforce; sex roles and practices; relationships and the institution of the family; health care; technology; and the investment marketplace. As a result, our society has given boomers more attention than any other group.

With all of this in mind, recreation professionals must understand that boomers will also redefine the leisure experience. Much of what is currently known about senior recreation values will be redefined under the boomer generation. Recreation professionals must use a different philosophical lens to learn about this generation—a lens that is focused on key values of this unique cohort:

- Boomers are concerned about chronic disease and have a desire to do whatever is possible to *postpone physical aging.*
- Boomers have *increasing amounts of discretionary money* as a result of escalating earning power, inheritances, and return on investments (this is true for many of them, but not all).
- Boomers will need support as they enter into an evident *new adult life* (retirement) with its own challenges and opportunities.
- Boomers are undergoing a psychological shift, from a desire to acquire material possessions toward *a desire to purchase enjoyable and satisfying experiences, particularly in leisure.*
- Boomers have a continued *absence of disposable time* due to complex lifestyles; however, their perspective on leisure *as a necessity* will remain.

Given these five key values, a wide range of opportunities awaits recreation professionals who anticipate and plan for the leisure challenges of the boomer cohort. Since we are only a few years away from the time the first boomer reaches age 65 (year 2011) but also know that many in the boomer generation are retiring soon, we need to know what makes boomers tick and what makes them unique—beyond simply their interests, what they like and do not like. Understanding what drives their interests comes from understanding their value system. An easy way to attain this understanding is to conduct a boomer assessment using tools such as the Cochran Baby Boomer Quiz.

Assess Your Agency's Preparedness

According to Dychtwald (2005, Home page), renowned psychologist, gerontologist, and founder of Age Wave in San Francisco, "It appears that boomer men and women are generally optimistic, innovative, and hopeful . . . and they're definitely gearing up for a new model of retirement." Age Wave is the nation's leader on population aging and can be found at www.agewave .com. Though there is much available information about boomers' lifestyles, in order to adequately address the onset of this large aging population, we as recreation professionals must ask ourselves and our agencies these three questions:

1. How well do we know boomers and their values?
2. Why do boomers participate in leisure?
3. Are we (I, my staff, and my agency) prepared for boomers?

We cannot adequately provide leisure programs or services without being internally prepared. The following three steps are designed to provide recreation professionals with an assessment tool for measuring both their individual and their agency's preparedness for boomers. Further, these steps support and encourage adoption of a boomer lens, using values to develop leisure programs for the baby boomer cohort.

1. Get to Know Boomers

Let's face it—until we understand the leisure values of the boomers, it will be hard to meet their expectations. Begin with assessing how well you know the leisure values of boomers by taking the Cochran Baby Boomer Quiz (CBBQ) presented in chapter 2. Nine or 10 correct answers indicates readiness for the boomers with a good working knowledge of boomers' values. Scores of 6 to 8 reflect some knowledge but suggest that it would not hurt to learn more. Scores of 5 or less indicate that increasing boomer knowledge is needed now.

Take the time to plan, develop, and administer a leisure value survey to your local boomer participants and residents. Knowledge gained from this assessment is your most valuable programming tool. It is essential to become familiar with boomers in terms of their culture, values, lifestyle, and economic levels. Ask questions that will address these elements. Use questions that grasp their interests. Try to avoid long checklists and open-ended questions, which may lead to nonresponse or a lack of truthfulness.

2. Understand Why Boomers Participate in Leisure

The foundation for providing leisure programs and services is an understanding of why participants attend, what they want, and what they need. The leisure value section of the CBBQ 1 can be a very useful tool. The questions are based on six value areas—competitive, educational, physiological, social, relaxation, and aesthetic. Results should give a good indication of which leisure values boomers from differing locations seek from leisure participation and thus provide guidance for designing and implementing leisure programs. Further, as a continuation of step 1, see how boomers respond, and compare their answers to the answers of agency staff in order to judge the adequacy of staff knowledge of programming for this cohort.

In terms of specific leisure activity interests, get out and ask boomers what they enjoy doing during their leisure. You can do this creatively through e-mail, postal mail and boomer ballots, Web sites, creative thinking bash events, interviews, and advisory committees. Whatever the case, if not asked directly, boomers will not tell you, resulting in the possible failure of leisure programs. Is that a risk you or your agency is willing to take?

3. Educate Staff and the Agency

The importance of becoming informed about the values of boomers in leisure is apparent. We have discussed strategies for obtaining this information. The results of surveys and the information-gathering process go beyond pretty graphs and statistical data. This information must be used to educate staff—even those who may not directly provide services. Within an agency, examination of the values of a cohort, along with current trends, must be regular, consistent, and ongoing. An interesting way to educate staff is to invite speakers from a variety of backgrounds to talk about the future of the city or region over the next 5 to 10 years. Speakers could include representatives from business, education, law enforcement, community development, and social services. Another way to educate staff is to use questions from part 2 of CBBQ 2 (see appendix). Then compare your responses with those of other recreation professionals in your agency or community to identify levels of preparedness.

If your staff and agency ratings are satisfactory, success with the boomer cohort is highly possible. If ratings are not satisfactory, you can use this assessment tool as a learning experience. Further, you can use the suggestions in the next section as a guide for raising your boomer knowledge.

Strategize for Boomer Programming, Marketing, and Implementation

After becoming familiar with boomer values and interests through survey and assessment, you can take these six steps to develop ideas and strategies for getting boomers involved in your leisure programs and services:

1. Redesign agency mission and goals
2. Create and maintain a focused program image
3. Make a boomer plan
4. Schedule facilities and programs
5. Advertise and market to boomers
6. Evaluate programs and agency

1. Redesign Agency Mission and Goals

Regardless of how you choose to specifically define it, an organization's mission relates to its values, philosophy, goals, guidelines, and inherent culture. A mission statement allows an agency to obtain a shared understanding of core accomplishments, as well as of what it will not accomplish. Baby boomers are distinct. Boomers need to learn, discover and experience, belong, and obtain fulfillment. Recreation agencies must consider either adopting new or modifying existing mission statements to meet the unique values and leisure interests of this cohort. Baby boomers are focused on active, educational, and fun activities, giving new meaning to everything they do in leisure (Cochran, 2005). The values identified through assessment should be reflected in the agency mission and philosophy. Here's an example:

> The Sullivan Recreation Department strives to meet the baby boomer leisure values and activity interests by projecting an active lifestyle image, providing relevant educational options, and inspiring volunteer opportunities. We are committed to enhancing the quality of life and personal growth of boomers through participation in traditional and innovative programming. We are committed to effectively using all available resources and to sustaining the confidence of those we serve.

Based on the mission statement, goals should support measures of achievement of the mission. Goals should be brief enough to remember, clear enough to be written down, and specific enough to be attainable. These are good examples of goals:

- To maximize the citizen involvement of boomers in the planning and development of recreation programs and services

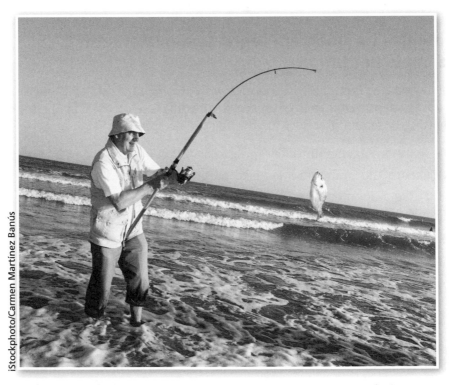

iStockphoto/Carmen Martinez Banús

Baby boomers will continue to participate in favorite pastimes during retirement. Recreational professionals must find ways to offer traditional activities while also spicing them up. Keep it interesting!

- To provide opportunities for boomers to contribute their knowledge and skills to the community
- To encourage the healthy and active lifestyles of boomers throughout all recreational programs

This step will allow agency staff to meet or exceed boomers' leisure values, needs, and expectations, as well as allow staff to be more prepared for the onset of boomers in leisure programs and recreation facilities.

2. Create and Maintain a Focused Program Image

Before you offer leisure programs to boomers, consider how your agency or program will appear to and be remembered by the boomers. In marketing terms, this image is your program "brand." As we have emphasized, boomers make up the largest share of the U.S. population. Boomers are a self-focused generation that has high expectations and demands quality services. With 76 million boomers in our aging society, a boomer program image or brand should be bold and energetic, reflecting the qualities of this population. A great image comes from a great imagination, teamwork, effort, time, willingness to change, and individual flexibility. Image is created and maintained, in part, by the following:

- Bringing together committed staff that are able to work with values and an energetic population
- Creating attractive facilities and grounds that can be used for competitive sports and active participant usage
- Implementing quality programs and programs that appropriately address a population of movers
- Developing an effective marketing program targeted toward the boomer cohort—one that defines styles, is filled with pizzazz, and has an adventurous flair
- Having an extraordinary customer service program that attracts and retains loyal boomer participants—boomers expect good service and will not be patient with the status quo

3. Make a Boomer Plan

With knowledge of boomer values, knowledge of why boomers participate in leisure, a values-focused mission and goals, and a focused program image, making a boomer plan is the next step. This plan should be realistic in terms of meeting the values and leisure interests of boomers, primarily focusing on leisure programs. Two concepts present themselves when you develop a boomer plan:

1. Based on the high education level of most boomers and their continued drive for learning, even in leisure, leisure activities and events should be meaningfully related to one another. For example, a nature program

might involve experiences in hiking, building shelter, education on edible plants, arts and crafts, creative writing, and games. All the experiences are richer and more meaningful as they converge rather than if they have been approached in a narrow fashion.

2. Leisure programs should involve challenge, continuity, and depth. Boomers thrive on these concepts. *Challenge* implies that the leisure program must provide activities that are new to people, test their skills, and heighten their motivation, thus expanding the recreational horizons of participants. *Continuity* means that the program provides activities that continue leisure skills and interests into an active lifestyle. It also means that a person may continue a hobby or recreational interest year after year, experiencing it in greater *depth* and gaining greater rewards and satisfactions.

4. Schedule Facilities and Programs

Recreation and park agencies need to develop a comprehensive schedule of programs that maximizes attendance and patron satisfaction. Many leisure programs are scheduled in fixed, unimaginative ways. Boomers live active lifestyles. Indications are they will not slow down as they near retirement. Recreation professionals must consider balance, impact, location, and timing when scheduling facilities and programs for this new cohort (Rossman & Schlatter, 2003):

• **Balance:** Avoid smultaneously scheduling similar activities that may appeal to the same target group. Schedule a balanced variety of leisure programs at any one time in order to maximize participation levels. For example, rather than four sport activities, try scheduling art, fitness, educational, and social activities—all of these are high enjoyment activities for boomers (Cochran, 2005).

• **Impact:** Many boomers are still raising children, so scheduling a major soccer match for a child at the same time as a backpacking trip for adults may not be appropriate to those who wish to participate in both events. Consider all elements that might be affected.

• **Location:** If the program is not conveniently located, participants may not attend due to lack of transportation or the amount of time it takes to get there. Access promotes use, so schedule programs that are easy to get to or provide transportation options to those who may need them. Because boomers are active, an idea that may work is to have participants meet at one location, then ride their bikes as a group to the actual event location. This would fit in with the healthy lifestyles that boomers lead and still permit conducting a program at an out-of-the-way location.

• **Timing:** When scheduling facilities or programs for boomer use, it is imperative to understand the personal schedules of typical boomers. Many boomers plan to work well beyond the usual retirement age. The boomer

Deb Smith

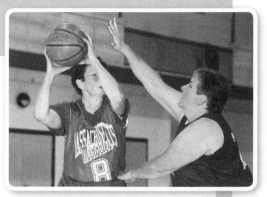

I've played basketball all my life. I love this game! About 15 years ago, I got connected with a group of 50-year-old women after one of them asked me if I would like to coach them. I wasn't 50 yet so I couldn't play, but I loved coaching this group of women. The players weren't very skilled but they would do anything I asked them to do. They worked hard in practice. They were all pre-Title IX so they had played only the modified game of basketball—you know, the game where you stay on your side of the court and I'll stay on my side of the court.

Along came the year 2004 and I was finally old enough to play on the senior women's basketball team. My team was named the Hot Flashes and we were pretty decent. My first National Senior Games as an athlete were in Pittsburg the summer of 2005. What a great time it was! We were on our way home waiting in the airport when a teammate and I looked at each other and said, "We need a basketball camp to go to." And shortly after this day I created Not Too Late Basketball Camp.

It was the summer of 2006 that I offered the first Not Too Late Basketball Camp. Fifty-three women from 13 states participated in this camp. It was a glorious weekend of basketball. All these women who had never really been coached and taught the game of basketball had the time of their lives. Area coaches worked with the athletes and showed them skills and drills, gave them positive feedback, and showed the utmost respect for the players. Likewise, the players were in awe of the respect that these younger coaches had for them. Over the years the camp has grown: We had 88 attendees from 19 states in 2008.

This camp is a dream come true for me. It's a challenge to become a better player, get in better shape, work together with my teammates toward a common goal, and be successful.

Profile and photo courtesy of Deb Smith.

cohort covers an 18-year span. Therefore we need to find out the answers to various questions: When are boomers at home? When are most of the boomers at work? Do boomers have children and after-school carpool commitments? Which days and times do boomers find convenient for programs or facility hours? Developing a balance of program and facility times takes practice and understanding of boomers' lifestyles. Creative use of facilities and resources will allow opportunities for each person to participate at times when he or she is able to do so.

5. Advertise and Market to Boomers

The boomer generation will not perceive leisure as within the same limits as the current older population. Boomers are outgoing and distinctive, and since their birth they have led the direction of society in terms of consumerism, culture, education, and economics. Consider the diversity of this group and implement those elements within your plan—ask what would attract them. To enhance visibility of your programs and increase participation, begin with advertising and promotion. These two elements work together and can often be the determining factor in success or failure of leisure programs. Advertising informs the marketplace about program activities, events, products, and services. Promotion takes the appropriate actions to sell the values and benefits of program activities, events, products, and services.

Get boomers involved in designing programs for themselves. Consider the diversity among boomers and implement advertising and marketing using these techniques:

- Get boomers involved now: Use their knowledge and expertise in designing and developing current programs, before you are faced with their resistance to traditional senior leisure programs, services, and facilities.
- Develop a campaign appealing to their interests. Be creative. Use a free drawing or a discount coupon incentive to encourage participation and registration of participants.
- Develop a link on your agency's Web site that targets the boomers' leisure values and activity interests.
- Design and distribute a newsletter specifically for active boomer adults in your community. Besides regular postal mail, try these methods: e-mail, various public facilities (such as the library, concert halls, and gourmet coffee shops), the Chamber of Commerce, key local businesses, and public transportation areas.
- Design and offer a strong adult leisure education program enabling boomers to enhance the quality of their lives through agency offerings. This will hopefully serve the boomer population into their senior years with minor modifications along the way.

Remember, when planning your advertising and publicity techniques, that the program itself is less important than the values and benefits of participating. Recreation professionals provide opportunities for people to access the endless benefits received from participation. Boomers are after the benefits derived from their leisure experiences.

6. Evaluate Programs and Agency

Many accept evaluation as a key element to program success; however, few actually evaluate fully and consistently. For programmers, evaluation is a learning tool. Do not just file evaluations away! Each program should reflect the agency's mission and goals, as well as the values of boomers. Is there a match between the agency and its program participants? Relying solely on attendance records is a mistake. Although this common method provides some accuracy with reference to participation numbers and can support budget requests, there are many questions that attendance figures do not answer: Did the participant enjoy the program? What could be improved? How can the program attract more participants? Does this program meet the goals and values intended? What is the potential for program growth?

Agencies want boomers to enjoy leisure experiences for a long time. Use multiple evaluation methods to ensure continued enjoyment:

- Adopt techniques that include evaluation before and after programs.
- Perform observations of programs.
- Establish written reports of lessons learned.
- Conduct informal interviews with staff and boomer participants.
- Hold open house nights and invite boomers to your facility for a preview of available programs and facilities, as well as to meet staff.

Practical application of these guidelines by professionals results in success, as these comments suggest:

- "Your program paradigm framework is a useful tool . . . assisting in the process and strategies to effectively engage staff to develop effective programming guidelines" (Barry Weiss, recreation director for the City of San Carlos, CA).
- "My staff and I find your information encouraging and reaffirming as we see success in the way our programs and our philosophy is changing in preparation for boomers" (Terry Hilton, Howard County, MD).

Recreation professionals will need to redefine the industry as boomers redefine retirement. The baby boomers were the dominant generation of the last half of the 20th century and continue to dominate today. As they march toward retirement, boomers are not going to be satisfied with a "regularly scheduled program" as seen in the typical senior center. The traditional approaches to leisure programming and use of leisure facilities will have to break from the norms to meet the demands of the baby boomer generation. Successful programming for this generation requires a new philosophy— looking at values through the boomer lens. Values can be assessed through a variety of tools, including the CBBQ.

You can put knowledge gained through such evaluations to use through a set of guiding principles. These include setting the boomer picture by knowing the characteristics of this cohort and understanding their values; using assessment tools to understand why boomers participate in leisure and to educate staff about this generation; and using a boomer lens to develop strategies for planning and implementing programs for boomers.

The guiding principles contribute to the body of knowledge available to recreation professionals charged with the responsibility of planning and providing leisure opportunities for the baby boomer cohort. These guidelines can instill confidence, creativity, and support for a values-based philosophical lens in leisure programming, not only for baby boomers but for any cohort.

5

Getting Groovy

· · · · · · · · · · · ·

Arts and Culture Program Ideas

On any given day, more people in the United States attend arts and culture events than attend sport events. Moreover, people who participate in the arts by listening to classical or jazz radio, attending or participating in a performing arts event, and reading literature are more likely to attend sporting events and volunteer their time and expertise in the community (National Endowment for the Arts, 2005).

The arts boom was fueled in the 1970s, a time when the boomers themselves were in their youth and early 20s. During this period the number of artists and art organizations, and support for public art as well as corporate and foundation philanthropy toward the arts, expanded enormously. Of the many who attended university, boomers were exposed to a variety of courses and degree options specifically in the arts. Boomers defined themselves by popular music, selecting genres with which to identify from the varied fare offered by local disk jockeys and also live in clubs and other commercial venues. Additionally, boomers grew up when television programming was developing. Television programming influenced their socialization with arts and cultural programs.

On the one hand, baby boomers came of age in a time of greater affluence; on the other, it was a time of becoming independent—an outcome of the Vietnam War. Artistic expression gave them an outlet to express their feelings of separation and identity. Given the sheer size of their cohort, boomers constituted a highly particularized audience of significant mass, and one that both political activists and the music industry could appeal to without any need for gaining broader popularity across generations.

Arts and culture activities enrich people's lives by providing meaning and stimulation. Social relationships are enhanced through sharing the experience of, discussing, or creating art. Such activities provide opportunities to build understanding and appreciation by increasing cooperation, tolerance, and recognition of the richness of diversity. Participation traditionally provides avenues of self-expression and identity formation, enhanced self-esteem, increased self-awareness, and improved creative thinking and problem-solving abilities. Arts and cultural activities provide overall improvement in the quality of life in the community at large. These outcomes are especially important to the baby boomer generation, who seek meaningful experiences.

As education and income increase, so does participation in the arts for all ages. With baby boomers as the most highly educated cohort ever, researchers have been surprised by a slight decline in participation in the arts after World War II. Even with this decline, a National Endowment for the Arts study showed that nearly 65 percent of boomers personally participated in 2002. Arts and cultural programs are rapidly growing in popularity at community centers for people ages 50 and older. A possible explanation may be that whereas time and money may be preempted by the activities of children who still live at home and by the demands of peak career experiences, these resources may become more available after children leave home or parents retire.

In any case, participation in the arts remains substantial and demand continues. According to a study conducted by the Institute for Innovation in Social Policy titled *Arts, Culture, and the Social Health of the Nation 2005* (Miringoff & Opdycke, 2005), people's favorite activities are as follows (in order of popularity):

- Listening to music
- Reading books
- Doing creative work
- Going to the movies
- Attending live performances
- Going to art shows or museums

Directly reflective of the interests of the baby boomers, The Police, Pink Floyd, Van Halen, Sting, The Rolling Stones, and The Eagles—each composed almost entirely of baby boomers—were among the top-grossing live performance tours of 2007.

Several ideas that may help recreation professionals plan and implement arts and culture programs for the boomers involve working with other agencies (Carpenter & Parr, 2005, p. 32):

- Collaborate with local arts organizations to plan and implement arts and cultural programs; collaborate with and hire local artists to facilitate community arts programs for boomers.
- Cooperate with local, regional, or state agencies to apply for grant funding to support cultural arts programs.

- Encourage university researchers who are studying the social and psychological benefits of arts participation to include your participants in their studies.

- Serve as a board member on local nonprofit arts organizations; encourage boomers who have arts experiences and skills to work with beginners.

MARKETING TIPS

Remember that even the most inspired and innovative programs in the world are worthless unless people know about them. If, in the past, your agency has been known mostly for its athletics and youth-based programs, you will have to work especially hard to reposition yourself as a creative arts, boomer-serving organization. Don't be disappointed if people don't immediately flock to your adult enrichment programs, since you are a relative newcomer to this marketplace.

As you're adding new programs to your inventory to better meet the needs of baby boomers, make sure you are also implementing new marketing and communication methods. Programs such as those listed in this chapter, which inspire creativity and bring out the artist within, especially call for innovative marketing messaging, graphics, and design. People will judge the quality of your programs based on the quality of your marketing. If your marketing is boring or dull, prospects may assume that your programs are boring or dull.

Ideas for Copy About Creative Art Programs

- Release the Artist Within
- Art Is Good for the Heart (see if you can cite a study that connects the benefits of participating in creative arts programs to stress reduction and heart health)
- What Do Picasso, Monet, Van Gogh, and YOU Have in Common?
- You're Invited to Have a Brush With Greatness
- Time to Mess Up!
- Life Can Be a Little Messy
- When Was the Last Time You Really Messed Up?

Remember to build relationships with gatekeepers who can lead you or introduce your programs to "hot prospects." Gatekeepers might also help you locate qualified instructors and promote your programs. If you are an agency with little or no studio space for creative arts programs, gatekeepers might offer the perfect solution by allowing you to bring your programs into their facilities.

Gatekeepers for Creative Arts Programs

- Art supply stores
- Craft stores

- Mental health care community; physical, occupational, and recreation therapists (art therapy is a growing field for people of all ages—not just children)
- School administrators and teachers (public, private, adult educators) looking for new ideas for classroom projects

ARTS AND CULTURE PROGRAM IDEAS

The programs described in this chapter offer a wide range of participation in the arts. Some programs are social, some are educational, and others allow individual expression. All of them exercise the brain.

ART SAMPLER

> **Description**

Try them all! Get a taste of various ways to express yourself through art. A different medium will be used each week: sketching, charcoal drawing, pen and ink drawing, cartooning, watercolor painting, acrylic painting, pottery (two weeks). Attend one or all. Optional art show at the end of the course.

> **Purpose and Goals**

* To be introduced to various media for art
* To gain a very brief background on the use of each medium
* To understand principles of using each medium

> **Length and Format**

Eight weeks, 2 hours per week

> **Space**

Varies according to the medium—check with instructor for each medium

> **Staffing**

Instructor for each class

> **Equipment and Materials**

* A materials list for each class
* Tables and chairs for all participants

> **Implementation**

1. If a different venue is used for each class, explicit information for participants will be essential. Include a schedule, addresses, and directions for each class along with a list of basic supplies needed and sources for the supplies.
2. Ask instructors to provide a brief background on the history of their medium, an introduction to supplies used, a list of resource books, and places where participants can go to see live examples of the medium on display.

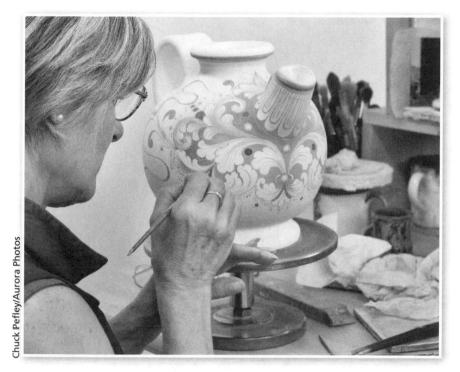

Chuck Pefley/Aurora Photos

Baby boomers are eager to either learn new skills or improve on ones they already know.

> *Options and Variations*

* Try partnering with community-based arts organizations, a local high school, or a local university for space and instructors. Graduate students are often looking for ways to gain experience teaching.

* Collaborate with local artists or artists' guilds to facilitate arts programs. Keep in mind that good artists are not always good instructors.

* A local arts supplies store may provide a discount for your students. Also, you may purchase supplies beyond the basics for students to share.

INTERNATIONAL FOOD

> *Description*

Ever wonder what *huaraches* or *borscht* tastes like? Or where to find a certain spice for an Indian recipe you have? Learn more about international foods, local markets, and tools for preparation.

> *Purpose and Goals*

* To be introduced to and learn about foods from different cultures
* To find out how to locate these foods
* To have a cultural experience

➤ *Length and Format*

Varied; one 2-hour session or multiple sessions—one for each type of food

➤ *Space*

Large room with tables and chairs

➤ *Staffing*

One facilitator, variety of guest speakers if available to introduce their cultures

➤ *Equipment and Materials*

* Packet including lists of local cultural restaurants and local cultural food markets, several international recipes, calendar of international fairs in the area, note cards, and a pen for taking notes
* Samples of several international foods or a luncheon in which international foods will be served
* Detailed PowerPoint presentation

➤ *Implementation*

1. Provide background on each culture and how the foods are served.
2. Provide a description of the nutritional values for each of these foods.
3. Provide a cultural experience with decorations and explanations of when and how the foods are served.

➤ *Options and Variations*

* The group can be divided into smaller groups, with participants choosing which culture or food to experience.
* A follow-up session can be provided on preparing some international foods.

ART FOR YOUR HEART!

➤ *Description*

Take a vacation for your spirit by painting your heart out! Whether you are a beginner or more advanced, enjoy the time to express yourself freely while learning or improving skills in color and design.

➤ *Purpose and Goals*

To learn how to paint with watercolors

➤ *Length and Format*

Three-day seminar

➤ *Space*

Facility with access to water

➤ *Staffing*

Various ratios according to instructor experience and participants' needs (cost for the course will cover materials, so the more participants, the lower the cost)

➤ *Equipment and Materials*

* Can either provide paints, paper, brushes, and so on, or provide participants with a list of materials needed prior to the beginning of class

* Photos that participants may bring for inspiration, or simply their own imaginations

➤ *Implementation*

1. Teach participants the basic techniques and rules for painting with watercolors.

2. Present examples of various watercolor artists' works (PowerPoint slide show, books from library).

3. Allow participants to create, and offer help and guidance when asked.

4. Display works in community center or town library for a week after class (for those who wish to display their work). Show members of the community what they can do in recreation programs.

➤ *Options and Variations*

Include several "discussion breaks" during which topics can be shared or discussed. Examples might be techniques that participants have found useful, understanding "modern" art, and brushing techniques, as well as questions like "What is creativity?" and "Where do you get your inspiration?"

> **Being an artist doesn't mean that you're a good artist. That was the bargain I first made with myself: I'd say, I'm an artist, but I'm not really very good.**
> —*Paul Simon*

BEGINNER'S FOLK GUITAR NIGHT

➤ *Description*

Do you miss hootenannies and folk songs? Always wanted to play guitar? Now's your chance to learn! The basics of chording and strumming will be taught in this class, using the folk songs we loved most while growing up.

➤ *Purpose and Goals*
  * To learn some basics of guitar
  * To have a musical group experience
  * To relive the days of youth

➤ *Length and Format*
A 2- to 3-hour workshop

➤ *Space*
Room for sound to resonate in the space

➤ *Staffing*
Various ratios according to instructor experience and participants' needs

➤ *Equipment and Materials*
  * Guitars (ask participants on registration form if they will be bringing their own)
  * Guitar picks
  * Guitar tablature
  * Practice instruction sheets for participants to take home
  * Refreshments

➤ *Implementation*
  1. Obtain small percussion instruments such as cymbals or tambourines for those who do not wish to play the guitar, or whose fingers get sore, and to achieve a greater effect.
  2. Arrange for a proficient guitar instructor or player who will teach a few chords and then be able to lead the group in playing songs and singing. This activity can be held in a multipurpose room or around a campfire; the level of ambience is up to you.
  3. Have the instructor lead the group through some basic chords; then participants can practice in small groups or alone. Provide refreshments to allow for more socializing. After a period of practice, have the instructor lead the group through basic folk songs reminiscent of the 1960s. Music stores sell books of songs by Peter, Paul, and Mary; Joan Baez; Ian and Sylvia; Woody Guthrie; and Judy Collins. Participants could bring suggestions for songs to the program.
  4. Finish the evening with the group's best songs; give awards for most improved player, most accomplished player, the player most suited to "keeping the day job," and so on. Have fun!

➤ *Options and Variations*
  * The activity can be offered in the typical six- or eight-week class format, as a morning or afternoon workshop, or as a series. In a series format, a specific topic could be covered at each class. For example, one session might cover holding the guitar and pick, strumming, a couple of chords, and finger exercises. Another session could cover specific chords and

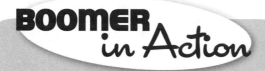

Buddy Parks

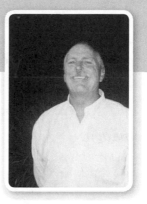

Who would have thought that typing my master's thesis at Louisiana State University would lead to a long-term hobby? I had written the thesis but needed someone to type it for me. With a firstborn child on the way, and little money for paying someone to type for me, I turned to my mother-in-law. She agreed to type for me in exchange for my refinishing an antique armoire that had been neglected for many years, laying in pieces in a workshed by my father-in-law's greenhouse. After digging out the most likely pieces and washing them off, I discovered side wood panels, a door, top and bottom pieces, and drawers for a project that I didn't know anything about.

I learned the art of refinishing old furniture the best way: by trial and error. I figured I could get the old paint and finishes removed simply by brushing on a stripping solution and using a scraper to get it off. Just two easy steps! I don't remember how many times I had to go to the hardware store and buy something else—something else, that is, that probably wouldn't work as claimed on the label. I had chemical burns on my fingers and stains on the carport of the house we were renting, and I killed substantial areas of the lawn. In reality, I had no idea what I was doing, but being both young and stubborn, I kept at it. Eventually, I had all the pieces stripped of their various coats.

Over time, I learned how to use sanders, steel wool, wood glue, and clamps to mend the cracks and make the wood look good. I had slowed down enough to pay attention to the detailed grooves, routed patterns, and intricate designs in each separate part. Then, after staining and sealing, I put all the pieces together. I was amazed by the outstanding look. My wife was amazed. My mother-in-law was so impressed, she paid a professional proofreader to review my paper and correct typos and grammatical errors.

Within a few weeks, my wife asked her mom about an antique dining room table that was in deplorable condition in the same shed by the same greenhouse. If I'd refinish it, it could be ours. Of course, I now had a fairly good knowledge of the task at hand, and the work was much easier. I also found a sense of personal satisfaction in the work and an appreciation for the piece of furniture. I was hooked on a hobby—not just refinishing an antique but finding a really beat-up and worthless antique and reworking it to something that any dealer would be proud to offer for sale.

Profile and photo courtesy of Buddy Parks.

how to make chord changes. Another might focus on picking and how to care for your instrument.

* A group "concert" can be held at the end of a workshop or class session.
* An outdoor venue with a campfire would add atmosphere; participants need to be seated close together.

FOREIGN FILMS

> *Description*

The rest of the world makes films different in content and style from our glitzy Hollywood fare. Come view human stories through different perspectives. Best films from international film festivals will be shown and discussed—a different country and genre each week during this series.

> *Purpose and Goals*

* To learn about films from other countries and perspectives
* To understand culture through film
* To share perspectives on messages conveyed through this medium

> *Length and Format*

Eight sessions, 2 to 2-1/2 hours each

> *Space*

Dark, quiet room with comfortable chairs

> *Staffing*

One person to introduce the film, show the film, and lead the discussion

> *Equipment and Materials*

Projector, film or DVD*

> *Implementation*

1. Introduce the film by establishing its credentials (director, country, plot synopsis, awards won and at which festivals), and point out aspects to observe during the showing.
2. Have a brief break with refreshments after the film; then lead discussion of plot, characters, setting, cultural aspects, and so on.

> *Options and Variations*

* A cinema studies professor or perhaps graduate students at a local university may be willing to lead the discussion.
* A panel of community members from the culture depicted in the film could lead a discussion following the film.
* Refreshments might include foods from the country in which the film was made.

*Check out the copyright for the film. Note that copyright on some films requires that you pay a fee to show the film even if you do not charge admission.

CELEBRATIONS AROUND THE WORLD

➤ *Description*

Like to celebrate? "Travel" around the world and celebrate occasions from across the globe.

➤ *Purpose and Goals*

* To be introduced to unfamiliar celebrations
* To broaden world perspectives
* To gain an understanding of other cultures

➤ *Length and Format*

About 2 hours

➤ *Space*

Depends on format

➤ *Staffing*

* Room host, registration staff if fee is involved
* Presenters (see "Options")

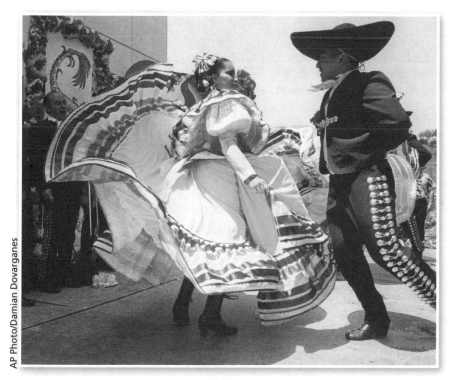

AP Photo/Damian Dovarganes

Baby boomers are eager to broaden their horizons. Seek out multicultural experiences in your area and incorporate a leisure activity into it.

> **Equipment and Materials**
>   * Optional (may be helpful): a "map" of the exhibit space
>   * Tables and chairs for guest presenters
>   * PowerPoint equipment, boom box, access to kitchen equipment (may be needed for guest presenters)

> **Implementation**
>
> If the activity is held in a "bazaar" or "fair" format, you will need to lay out foot traffic pattern flow and possible performance area.

> **Options and Variations**
>   * A local university may be a good source for exhibitors. The activity may be done as part of a university class (English as a second language, multicultural issues, world religions, geography, or history).
>   * Native costumes, flags, artifacts, and information sheets should be encouraged.
>   * For more in-depth information and discussion, a series of presentations, with a focus on one culture at a time, is an alternative to having multiple exhibits.

INDIE FARE: OFF-THE-GRID FILMS

> **Description**
>
> Tired of the same old formulaic Hollywood glitz? Come see the indies that everyone is talking about. A different independent film will be shown each week, followed by discussion.

> **Purpose and Goals**
>   * To view artistic films with real content
>   * To explore the human condition through film

> **Length and Format**
>
> Each showing 2 to 2-1/2 hours

> **Space**
>
> Dark, quiet room with comfortable chairs

> **Staffing**
>
> One person to preview the film, show it, and lead discussion

> **Equipment and Materials**
>
> Film or DVD*, liner notes, critics' reviews

> **Implementation**
>
> Preview the film (director, source material, shooting locations, plot intricacies, and so on). After showing the film, have a break—preferably with refreshments. Lead a discussion (overall impressions, plot message, aspects of the plot, acting, setting, music, similarities to the book [if based on a book], and so on).

> *Options and Variations*

The sessions could be based on themes. Examples:

* "Films of the Heart" or "Presidents on Parade" in February for Valentine's Day or Presidents' Day
* "Patriots Arise" for Fourth of July
* "Working Wisdom" for Labor Day in September

*Check out the copyright for the film. Note that copyright on some films requires that you pay a fee to show the film even if you do not charge admission.

LEARN AN INSTRUMENT

> *Description*

Have you ever wanted to play a clarinet? A French horn? A cello? Here's your chance to sample these instruments. You will sample each "family" of instruments. You will explore the features of each instrument in the family, how it is played, and great music composed for that instrument.

> *Purpose and Goals*

* To learn what each major instrument in each family of instruments can and cannot do
* To try out each instrument
* To explore music that features each family of instruments and individual instruments within the family

> *Length and Format*

Three 2-hour sessions for each family of instruments

> *Space*

Space where the "music" will not bother other concurrent classes

> *Staffing*

Depends on the instrument

> *Equipment and Materials*

Sample instruments

> *Implementation*

1. Only one family of instruments should be taught at a time. For example, during the string family classes, violin, viola, cello, and bass may be taught during one class; banjo and mandolin in the second class; and guitar and harp in the third class.

2. Each class should include a demonstration of the features and parts of each instrument, listening to great pieces of music that feature the instrument, instruction in how to play it, and time for participants to actually play the instrument themselves. Some instruments can be shared if each participant is provided with his or her own mouthpiece; mouthpieces can be attached to the instrument as it is passed around.

3. This may be a good summer class, as music stores are more likely to have rental instruments available when school is not in session.

> *Options and Variations*

A local high school or music store may be willing to provide sample instruments and instruction. Also graduate students in music programs in a nearby university may be willing to teach the classes. Participants may also enjoy giving a simple "concert" (using a short, easy tune such as "Happy Birthday") at the end of each class.

CREATING DESIGNS

> *Description*

Each session is themed and will use craft, decoration, and entertainment ideas from crafters' Web sites.

> *Purpose and Goals*
  * To get together for socialization
  * To have creative expression stimulated
  * To learn something new

> *Length and Format*

A series of 2- or 3-hour sessions

> *Space*

Multipurpose room

> *Staffing*

One to three staff, depending on the complexity of the project

> *Equipment and Materials*

Depend on crafts being made or activities being done (see "Options" section for ideas)

> *Implementation*

To prepare, choose a theme and research activities at www.marthastewart .com or your local craft shop. Require preregistration so you can create an accurate supplies order. Provide refreshments.

> *Options and Variations*
  * Sample theme: The Perfect Picnic! The activities for this 150-minute session are Paper Plate Update, Food Flags, Balloon Fireworks, and Origami Picnic Basket. Refreshments to be served: brownies displayed on the updated paper plates, finger sandwiches held together with food flags, and a sparkling fruit punch.
  * Themes can be seasonal: Examples are summer picnics, going to the beach, using fall colors, or beating the winter doldrums. Themes can stimulate creative ways of making special days more special, such as a

winter solstice or Presidents' Day celebration. Special occasions can also create themes. You could celebrate famous people's birthdays (Oprah Winfrey's or Gloria Steinham's) or have an event called "[insert the name of your town] Celebrates Mary Jones' 50th Birthday." Occasions that have the potential to elicit mixed feelings can also be spiced up with celebratory fun (for example, a last-child-leaving-home mini-festival).

MAKE YOUR OWN MOVIE

> ### Description

Do you fantasize about directing the perfect movie? Have a story you want to tell? Learn how to make your own home-grown movie with Hollywood appeal.

> ### Purpose and Goals

* To explore a form of self-expression and creativity
* To learn the process of movie making
* To get hands-on experience with storyboards, casting, taping, directing, and editing movies

> ### Length and Format

Depend on the instructor and class size (the instructor can tell you the length of each class and the number of weeks)

> ### Space

* Classroom space
* Access to editing and viewing equipment and rooms (later in the course)

> ### Staffing

One instructor

> ### Equipment and Materials

Handouts, film, cameras, projector, editing equipment

> ### Implementation

The film instructor should have a week-by-week lesson plan and assignments, as well as consultation time outside class. Class and instructor critique of participants' work should be included.

> ### Options and Variations

* Film studies professors or graduate students or local access television staff could instruct the class.
* Local access television studio facilities and time are usually set aside for public use.
* Final films may be aired on the local access television station, or an event at the community center might be held to show the best films (good advertisement for the next class).

SPICE UP THE SALSA

> **Description**

Salsa is a fun, easy-to-learn, social dance. It can be on the sedate side or very spicy. No partner necessary. Chips and salsa samples included.

> **Purpose and Goals**

* To learn a popular dance style
* To understand the role of dance in culture
* To get some exercise in a social, fun environment

> **Length and Format**

Series of sessions 1-1/2 to 2 hours each

> **Space**

Room with space to dance and also comfortable seating

> **Staffing**

One or two instructors

> **Equipment and Materials**

Salsa music, loudspeakers, cordless microphone (if the number of participants is large)

> **Implementation**

1. At the first session, you can show a DVD that illustrates types of salsa dance movements and steps. Each week you can preview the next session's lesson.

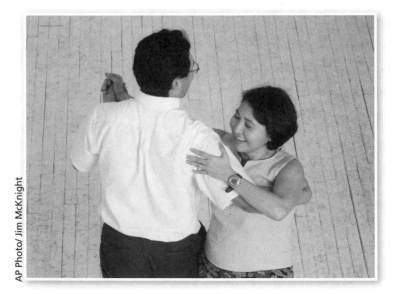

AP Photo/ Jim McKnight

Dancing is a great way to combine physical activity and fun.

2. A salsa dance, complete with decorations and costumes (if desired), could make a good culminating activity.

➤ *Options and Variations*

To add interest, a local Mexican restaurant could provide chips and a sampler of salsa.

SILENT FILM

➤ *Description*

The silent film era was an exciting time in the history of film. Learn how this genre came about. See the first-ever silent film. Learn how these films were made, and learn about the artists who made them.

➤ *Purpose and Goals*

* To understand the silent film genre
* To review exemplary silent films
* To learn how silent film was created
* To understand the role of music in these films

➤ *Length and Format*

Series of sessions 1-1/2 to 2 hours each

➤ *Space*

Dark, quiet room with comfortable seating

➤ *Staffing*

One person to preview the film, show it, and discuss its features

➤ *Equipment and Materials*

Projector and films*

➤ *Implementation*

1. At the first session, a mini-"lecture" on silent film history should be provided. Then *Birth of a Nation* should be shown. Because of its controversial subject matter, this film is sure to generate a serious discussion of the film's features. A preview of the next session's film should be presented each week.

2. At each subsequent session, information about the film itself, director, actors, features, and so on should be given before the film is shown.

➤ *Options and Variations*

* Different genres can be shown each week (for example, "horror" films such as *Nosferatu,* the first vampire film). Different actors can be featured such as Charlie Chaplin.

* Also, there is a resurgence of orchestras and individual musicians that provide live music for showings of silent films. An orchestra member or other musician might be willing to talk about the original scores, how the music is timed with the film, and so on.

*Check the copyright. You may have to pay a fee to show the film even if you do not charge admission.

OPERA OVER EASY

> **Description**

Have you always wondered what people see in opera? Find out what draws them to this art form, how opera is developed, what makes a good story line, and how the music progresses.

> **Purpose**

* To develop an understanding of opera as an art form
* To explore the role of music, costume, and setting in furthering plots
* To compare operatic forms

> **Length and Format**

Four meetings, 1-1/2 hours each (followed by attending a performance)

> **Space**

Quiet room with space for participants to sit and see a screen

> **Staffing**

One instructor

> **Equipment and Materials**

Projector, DVDs of various operatic forms, handouts of terms with their definitions

> **Implementation**

1. Start with light opera before moving to the "heavy-duty" forms. Show a DVD documentary on the making of an opera. Discuss aspects of production: singers, music, costuming, set design, production crew, lighting.
2. End the class with a trip to see a live opera, followed by a discussion (perhaps at a restaurant) immediately after the performance.

> **Options and Variations**

* Have guest speakers from an opera production company (director, orchestra conductor, featured opera singers, sound and light director).
* Arrange for a behind-the-scenes tour.
* Arrange for participants to meet the cast backstage.
* One class might consist of helping to build or paint sets.

WOMEN IN THE DIRECTOR'S CHAIR

> **Description**

An increasing number of women are taking the director's seat and producing top-quality movies. Preview two of these films and talk with the director before and after the viewing.

➤ *Purpose and Goals*
  * To be introduced to women as a strong force in movie making
  * To gain insight into the making of films
  * To better understand the role of the director
  * To share ideas about films and filmmaking

➤ *Length and Format*
Two meetings, about 3 hours each

➤ *Space*
Large, dark, quiet room with comfortable seating

➤ *Staffing*
Person to introduce the speaker(s), also ticket takers if admission is charged

➤ *Equipment and Materials*
  * Film*
  * Popcorn!
  * Projector and audio speakers
  * Possibly table and chairs for discussion

➤ *Implementation*
Good instruction is needed to start the event. Set ground rules for discussion after the film.

➤ *Options and Variations*
  * You may want to offer snacks.
  * A local university or high school may be willing to cosponsor this event, provide auditorium space, or both.
  * The local or regional arts council may provide funds to help pay for the director's transportation or fee or for film rental.
  * You can add a discussion panel (e.g., local organization leaders, especially if topic is controversial; university professors; film critic).

*Check the copyright. You may have to pay a fee to show the film even if you do not charge admission.

WORLD CULTURES WORKSHOP AND FESTIVAL

➤ *Description*
Share the celebrations of the world. Learn about celebrations in other countries—and your own! Learn how to display aspects of cultural celebrations and present them at a family cross-cultural festival.

> *Purpose and Goals*
  * To learn about celebrations of other countries and ethnic groups
  * To learn how to share cultural experiences
  * To celebrate the richness of our differences and similarities

> *Length and Format*
One 2-hour workshop, one community festival

> *Space*
Meeting room for workshop; large space such as community or school gymnasium or park (if weather permits)

> *Staffing*
One staffperson to teach visual display techniques and give verbal presentation at the workshop, festival staff as needed

> *Equipment and Materials*
  * Artifacts brought by participants
  * Demonstration materials needed by instructor, who will show how to display various artifacts (flags, videos, posters, material arts, books, photos, toys, and so on)

> *Implementation*
  1. At the workshop, demonstrate how to display various artifacts so as to preserve them and keep them safe from public handling. Demonstrate how to label artifacts and ways to verbally present them.
  2. At the festival, each class participant should have a table and wall space (or cardboard, standup backing) for her or his display and should staff the display so that information can be conveyed and questions answered. The festival can be a family event open to the public.

> *Options and Variations*
Entertainment can be provided:
  * Dance demonstrations: Potential sources are dance class instructors (salsa, belly dance, country two-step, square dance club, university folk dance classes, Scottish country dancers, mummers, Highland dancers, Korean community church, and so on), university student organizations (Asian student organization, Indian student organization, French house, German house, and so on).
  * Art displays: Potential sources are fine arts museum, university, art gallery, foreign food restaurant owners, Greek Orthodox Church members, international student organizations on campuses.
  * Music: Potential sources are library international music section, university classes or student groups.

WORLD RELIGIONS

> *Description*

Throughout history, many religions have developed followers around the world. Learn how these religions got started, the beliefs and practices that attract followers, and the similarities and differences among world religions.

> *Purpose and Goals*

* To learn the major tenets of religions of the world
* To understand the similarities across world religions
* To appreciate the differences among world religions

> *Length and Format*

Series of classes 1-1/2 hours each—as many as the number of religions you want to cover

> *Space*

Quiet room with tables and chairs

> *Staffing*

Discussion leader

> *Equipment and Materials*

A reading packet for each registrant

> *Implementation*

Make it clear at the outset that the purpose is not to argue the merits or perceived faults in religious beliefs but to understand the foundations of those beliefs. Present and discuss the major tenets of each of the major religions in the world: basis for the religion (history), basic principles, beliefs, significance of major celebrations, similarities and differences among the major religions, similarities and differences among sects with the same religion (for example, Roman Catholics, Baptists, Anglicans, Presbyterians, Congregationalists, and Methodists within Christianity). Keep lecture to a minimum, using it only as a foundation for discussion.

> *Options and Variations*

* Community leaders in each religion could be guest speakers, discussants, or discussion leaders. University professors who teach religion courses could be speakers, discussants, or discussion leaders.
* A cross-religion panel discussion could be held at the end of the course.

6

Pursuing Pathways
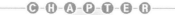
Education Program Ideas

Program planners have an advantage with baby boomers when developing education programs because of the high level of education this generation has achieved. Nearly 90 percent of boomers completed high school, and more than one-quarter (28.5 percent) obtained a bachelor's degree or higher (U.S. Census Bureau, 2000). Not only do they already value education, they are looking forward to pursuing more after retirement!

Strong rationale for including education programs in recreation program offerings comes from research on the brain and lifelong learning. Continuing to use the brain has implications for memory and recall. Moreover, education in later life has a direct relationship to health and well-being. Compared to people who don't continue to learn, those who do keep learning report themselves to be healthier and happier. Learning does not have to be in a formal classroom setting. In fact, many boomers prefer hands-on learning "in the field." Educational programs can take place wherever new information can be acquired—on a nature walk, in a farmer's field, in a kitchen, on a lake, or even on the sidewalk in front of your facility.

The best learning takes place when students of any age can apply the information to their daily lives within three days of the learning event. It is essential, then, that resources and supplies be readily available to participants. Program leaders do not necessarily have to give those supplies to participants, but a list of things to buy or places to purchase needed equipment and supplies should be a part of the learning experience. For example, if you offer a class on wine making from a kit, a list of retail suppliers should be handed out or available online. In addition, a list of resources for further information will allow the participants to learn even more.

Learning takes place in a variety of formats. In educating their students, medical schools follow a modified experiential education model:

"observe—do—teach." Recreation providers who already subscribe to an experiential education model in youth programs would do well to implement this model with baby boomers. This generation has already honed a lot of the "observe—do" part and can be called upon to exercise their brains with the "teach" part of the model.

Nearly half (47 percent) of baby boomers in the United States say they plan to spend more time volunteering during retirement (Thornhill & Martin, 2007). They can use their skills as teachers or facilitators for classes and workshops, as committee members for events and programs, as board members, as consultants, and in other volunteer capacities. Many park and recreation departments and other community agencies organize and manage job and volunteer placements for adolescents. Similar programs could be implemented for baby boomers in order to put their life skills to use. In the process of teaching someone else, we ourselves learn.

MARKETING PROGRAMS THAT PROMOTE BRAIN POWER

When it comes to marketing education programs, seminars, or workshops to baby boomers, keep in mind that you may be competing with centuries-old universities and other higher education institutions. In addition, many communities have long-standing adult education programs run by community learning centers or nonprofit or for-profit organizations. Rather than compete head-on, look for ways to fill gaps and partner with successful programs.

There are many "gatekeepers" that can help you connect to baby boomers who may be looking to increase their skills, brain power, or knowledge. Consider contacting people in the following areas:

• **Health care community:** The health care community is committed to both the physical and emotional health of patients. Studies show that playing games and doing puzzles can "exercise the brain" and may even reduce memory loss, reduce stress, and promote good mental health. Discuss program ideas with those specializing in Alzheimer's, Parkinson's disease, and dementia, as well as others in the medical field.

• **Travel agencies:** Boomers often look to travel agents to arrange vacations through organizations such as Elderhostel that focus on travel education. However, these trips can be very costly. Your agency may be able to offer local learning at a fraction of the cost.

• **Universities:** Universities have long been adjusting their operations, schedules, and products to meet the diverse needs and interests of students no matter what their age. Rather than competing head-on with existing university programs, look for ways to partner and to cross-promote or share resources.

- **Game and toy retailers:** These shop owners, whether online or in actual stores, attract all types of customers who are shopping for children or grandchildren. Help these retailers increase their sales by suggesting that they also market their products and games to adults. Together you can promote and host adult-only game nights or tournaments.

- **Game clubs:** A quick search on the Internet will help you discover local game clubs dedicated to just about any game you could possibly imagine. Even Yale, Notre Dame, and Ohio State University have Scrabble clubs that meet regularly.

Think beyond traditional "senior center games" such as bingo and bridge. Talk to retailers to find out what new and traditional games are hot. The list might include old and new games such as Bunco, Yahtzee, bingo, backgammon, chess, cribbage, Sudoku, and many more. Keep in mind that game enthusiasts not only play together but also love to compete and even travel together to out-of-town events. Connect to these groups to learn how you can support their passions and help attract more boomers to their clubs.

When developing a marketing strategy for any new set of programs, don't be afraid to aggressively and creatively spread the word. Boomers may actively look for mind-expanding programs to maintain or improve brain function, but may not realize that you offer options—especially if you are new to boomer-focused programs such as these. Improve your reach by working with, rather than against, other institutions, businesses, and groups already established as credible resources for adult education.

EDUCATION PROGRAM IDEAS

Baby boomers' recreation needs and interests are dictated more by their stage in life than by their age. Many factors enter into the equation, including time, money, caring for children who are still at home or who have come back home as adults to live, caring for aging parents, health status, and social group. Thus, it is difficult to predict that a certain set of activities will be more appropriate for "early," "middle," or "late" boomers. What *is* known is that at any life stage, the "use it or lose it" adage is applicable—and even more so with aging brains. Therefore, including a learning component in most if not all recreation programs is an advantage to the participant.

The remainder of this chapter presents descriptions of many different types of educational programs. Included is information on the latest technology for communications that will help keep boomers connected with younger generations (such as their children and grandchildren) and technology for their own entertainment. Educational programs with social components that will address life stage issues, such as healthy eating and cooking for two, are included. All of the programs include brain exercise, but some are designed specifically for that purpose.

INSTANT MESSENGER

➤ *Description*

Ever want to ask a friend a question without having to call on the phone, or want to have a chat via the Internet? Learn how with instant messenger.

➤ *Purpose and Goals*

* To obtain information about the benefits of technology
* To have a social experience
* To gain knowledge on using a different program to communicate

➤ *Length and Format*

One 2-hour session

➤ *Space*

Computer technology room

➤ *Staffing*

One facilitator

➤ *Equipment and Materials*

* Handouts on information covered in program
* Personal computers
* Internet hookup
* Large overhead screen

➤ *Implementation*

1. Provide an overview of benefits of an instant messenger (IM) account and the procedure for setting up an account.
2. Guide participants through creating a personal account.
3. Assist participants in practicing their new knowledge during the session, using each other for chatting through IM.

➤ *Options and Variations*

* Partners can work together if the number of computers is limited.
* If Internet is not available, participants will be provided the basics without a hands-on experience and will be given detailed written instructions.

COOKING FOR TWO

➤ *Description*

The kids have left home, and now it's just the two of you. Learn how to modify your techniques to cook for two. Tips for economical shopping and preparation of delicious, healthy meals for two people will be presented.

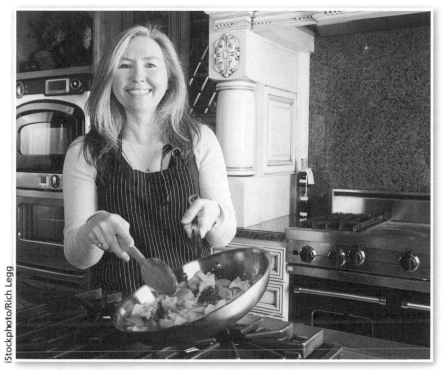

iStockphoto/Rich Legg

Baby boomers love to get adventurous in the kitchen. Offer different types of cooking classes to satisfy all tastes, from traditional to exotic.

➤ *Purpose and Goals*
   * To learn how to modify old shopping and cooking habits
   * To determine the right quantities of food to buy
   * To learn how to make food purchases for more than one meal
   * To collect healthy, delicious recipes for two people

➤ *Length and Format*
   One session, 1-1/2 to 2 hours

➤ *Space*
   Kitchen facility with room for participants to observe and work

➤ *Staffing*
   Instructor

➤ *Equipment and Materials*
   * Food
   * Cooking utensils (measuring cups, pots and pans, spoons, spatulas, whisks, measuring spoons, and so on)
   * Range-top, conventional oven, and microwave oven

> *Implementation*

1. Include information on selecting fruit, vegetables, and meats that can be used for more than one meal.
2. Give the educational information first, followed by demonstration and then participatory hands-on. Be sure to provide recipes for participants to take home.

> *Options and Variations*

* The local high school may have classroom cooking facilities available to the public (using the cooking arts teacher as the instructor may facilitate this arrangement). Other options include cooking facilities in a community center, senior center, or church.
* Several classes can be held, each with a theme: vegetarian dishes for two, beef night, chicken chow, vegetable side dishes, one-dish meals.
* The key for value-conscious boomers is to demonstrate how several different-tasting meals can be prepared from the same core ingredients with a few changes or additions, various methods of preparation, and varying herbs and spices.

EBAY

> *Description*

Looking for a certain gift, one that you can't find in stores? Need to sell something that you can't use any more? Learn how to use eBay and shop on the Web.

> *Purpose and Goals*

* To learn how eBay works
* To use eBay hands-on
* To experience a form of technology
* To become aware of risks involved with online selling and buying

> *Length and Format*

One 2-hour session

> *Space*

Room with Internet access

> *Staffing*

One facilitator

> *Equipment and Materials*

* Personal computers
* Large overhead screen on which the facilitator's computer can be projected
* Individual handouts on the program being demonstrated

➤ *Implementation*

1. Provide an overview of eBay.
2. Teach participants how to access and use eBay.
3. Assist participants in practicing and troubleshooting any difficulties with eBay.
4. List potential risks and how to minimize those risks.
5. Answer questions.

➤ *Options and Variations*

Participants can attend additional sessions in which they learn how to buy and sell merchandise. Participants need to be aware of risks and potential fraud and of ways to protect themselves. Specifics that should be addressed are charge-backs, PayPal, unconfirmed addresses, feedback scores, international shipping, rush shipping, checking out a new seller, paying to an address different from the shipping address, and other potential traps.

EXCEL FOR THE HOUSEHOLD

➤ *Description*

Get organized for carpooling, paying bills, running errands, and doing chores. Learn how to create and use an Excel spreadsheet to make your home life easier.

➤ *Purpose and Goals*

* To learn the uses of Excel
* To learn and apply the layout and maintenance of a spreadsheet
* To learn to apply the use of Excel in the home

➤ *Length and Format*

One 2-hour session

➤ *Space*

* Large room (computer technology room would work well)

➤ *Staffing*

One facilitator and one or more assistants to help participants individually

➤ *Equipment and Materials*

* Personal computers
* Printers
* Large overhead screen, visible to the whole room, that can be hooked up to the computer

> *Implementation*
>
> 1. Discuss the value of learning Excel.
> 2. Provide instructions for Excel.
> 3. Provide examples of Excel spreadsheets relevant to home use.
> 4. Give step-by-step instructions for creating a personal Excel sheet.

> *Options and Variations*

After participants create a spreadsheet they can print it off or save it to a scan disk for further use.

> **Never trust a computer you can't throw out a window.**
>
> —*Steve Wozniak, cofounder of Apple*

FACEBOOK FOR ALL AGES

> *Description*

Ever want to learn how to find old classmates or send a mass e-mail to bunches of friends? Learn about the new Web craze, Facebook. Find friends and keep in touch.

> *Purpose and Goals*
>
> * To learn how to use Facebook
> * To create a Facebook account
> * To gain access to a new social environment
> * To have a technology experience

> *Length and Format*

One 2-hour session

> *Space*

A room with personal computer hookup; one overhead screen needed

> *Staffing*

One facilitator

> *Equipment and Materials*
>
> * Handouts for instruction on Facebook
> * Personal computers with one hooked up to project onto screen
> * Overhead screen

➤ *Implementation*
1. Provide a handbook for instructions.
2. Show participants how to access the Facebook Web site.
3. Demonstrate sample sites.
4. Create an account with participants.
5. Discuss Facebook etiquette.
6. Assist participants in finding classmates or old friends.

MAKING SENSE OF NUTRITION LABELS ON FOODS

➤ *Description*

Ever wonder what maltitol or sorbitate is? Are they harmful? Do you know whether polyunsaturated, saturated, or trans fat is best for you? Learn how to read and interpret food labels to make healthy choices.

➤ *Purpose and Goals*
* To learn about food labels
* To apply knowledge to your own food choices
* To learn about nutrition and the nutritional values of various foods

➤ *Length and Format*

Varying; one or two 2-hour sessions

➤ *Space*

A large room with tables and chairs

➤ *Staffing*

One facilitator

➤ *Equipment and Materials*
* Paper and pens
* PowerPoint presentation on food labels, or overheads
* Examples of food labels, with specifics highlighted (e.g., fat calories, sugar calories)
* Overhead projection equipment
* Handout on definition of terms

➤ *Implementation*
1. Provide a background on population-specific nutrition.
2. Provide examples of food labels with highlighted categories—use both healthy and nonhealthy examples.
3. Provide a list of healthy food choices based on labels.

> *Options and Variations*
  * If two sessions are held, participants can bring in food labels during the second session and decipher ingredients.
  * Use group work to analyze food labels.
  * A nutritionist from a local hospital or a nutrition instructor from a local university may serve as facilitator.

FAST, HEALTHY MEALS

> *Description*

Need ideas for quick, healthy meals? Learn how to shop for, prepare, and enjoy quick meals.

> *Purpose and Goals*
  * To obtain nutritional information about several meals
  * To obtain multiple recipes for quick and healthy meals
  * To learn about healthy eating and meal preparation choices

> *Length and Format*

One 3-hour session

> *Space*

Large room with student work tables and front area for kitchen setup and teacher instruction area

> *Staffing*

One facilitator

> *Equipment and Materials*
  * Copies of all recipes used in the presentation
  * Meal preparation materials, ingredients, cooking tools
  * Nutritional chart information, PowerPoint style
  * PowerPoint presentation: computer, data projector, screen
  * Kitchen setup: stove, sink, oven, utensils

> *Implementation*
  1. Provide nutritional information.
  2. Provide a list of healthy choice ingredients.
  3. Demonstrate preparation of several healthy choice meals.
  4. Invite participants to sample the meals.

> *Options and Variations*
  * Stations can be set up for participants to prepare meals.
  * Overheads and handouts can be used instead of PowerPoint.

HOME WINE MAKING

> *Description*

Blueberries, grapes, and peaches (or even dandelions), oh my! Want to turn them into a fine beverage? Learn how to select and use the needed equipment, how to select and prepare the fruit, and how to make the wine step by step. Learn terms that will help you know what to ask about when you purchase equipment and ingredients.

> *Purpose and Goals*

* To learn the basics of making wine at home
* To learn appropriate terms to use in purchasing wine-making equipment and fruit

> *Length and Format*

One 2-hour session

> *Space*

Classroom

> *Staffing*

One instructor

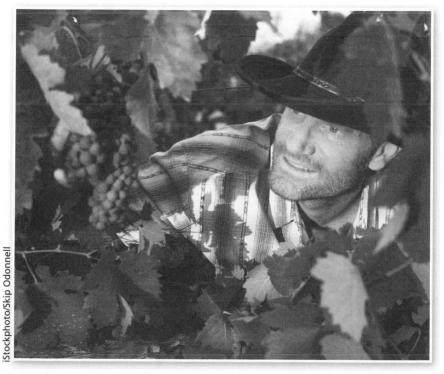

iStockphoto/Skip Odonnell

Wine making is a popular activity. Cover all the steps from grape to glass.

> *Equipment and Materials*
  * Wine-making equipment
  * Fruit and other wine ingredients

> *Implementation*
  1. Teach the terms participants need to know in order to purchase their wine-making equipment.
  2. Give tips and hints on finding a reputable equipment vendor and staying within a budget (when you should pay the extra for a higher-line product and when you can get by with the less expensive version).
  3. Hand out recipes for different kinds of wine, as well as step-by-step instructions.

> *Options and Variations*
  * A wine tasting could be held at the conclusion of the class.
  * Local wine-making equipment shop owners or wine aficionado club members may serve as instructors.

PAMPERED PETS

> *Description*

Pets provide us with a lot of entertainment and maybe even affection. Learn proper or new ways to take care of your special friend: grooming, making healthy foods, encouraging exercise and play. Know when to take your ailing pet to the vet and when to treat her at home (Did you know, for example, that you should not give chocolate or acetaminophen to dogs?).

> *Purpose and Goals*
  * To learn grooming techniques
  * To explore alternative, healthy foods for pets
  * To learn proper ways to exercise and play with pets
  * To know the signs and symptoms that require medical attention

> *Length and Format*

Four classes, 1-1/2 hours each (one each on grooming, healthy foods, exercise and play, and "How do I know when to take my pet to the vet?")

> *Space*

Room large enough to have pets out of cages and separated from each other

> *Staffing*

One knowledgeable instructor per class

> *Equipment and Materials*
>   * Grooming tools for demonstration
>   * Handouts on preparing homemade foods for pets

> *Implementation*
> An expert should lead each class.

> *Options and Variations*
>   * Include a liability waiver and a statement that the pet owner or registrant will keep control of his or her pet at all times.
>   * We advise segregating types of pets. For example, separate classes could be held for reptiles and amphibians, fish, birds, cats, dogs, and rodents.
>   * A holistic veterinarian could be the instructor for the healthy foods class and present information on how to make daily food and treats.
>   * A veterinarian should instruct the class on how to know that a pet needs to see the vet, the pros and cons of vaccinations, safe home medications, and so on. Pet groomers may teach the grooming class.
>   * Animal handlers (perhaps a reptilian biologist for snakes or a member of the local ferret club) can give proper instruction on exercise and play. An explanation of physiology and metabolism should be included.

PHILOSOPHERS' CAFÉ

> *Description*
> Do you enjoy discussing ideas over that morning cup of coffee or tea? Join other "philosophers" to discuss weekly themes.

> *Purpose and Goals*
>   * To explore ideas with others who have similar interests
>   * To learn about topics of interest
>   * To socialize
>   * To have intellectual discussions

> *Length*
> One or two hours per week; same time, same place each week

> *Space*
> Room with tables and comfortable chairs

> *Staffing*
> One facilitator whose job is to make sure everyone has a chance to speak and who asks questions to keep the discussion flowing

> *Materials*
> Coffee and tea

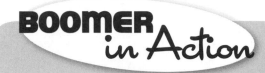

Ernie Noa

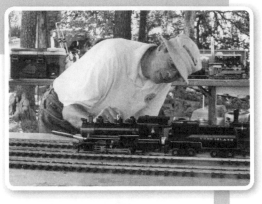

I must have been 6 years old when my dad gave me an American Flyer train set for Christmas. I think he had a secret desire to play with the train set, being from the Depression era. So my interests in trains started at a very early age. I also always had the desire to tinker with mechanical things.

Fast-forward to the 1990s, and my interest reignited with miniature live steam engines in gauge one (45 mm gauge). I had been building a garden railroad and wanted a steam engine to pull some cars I had built. At the time most everything was plastic, expensive, and of very poor quality. So I thought I could build an engine myself. One thing led to another and the decision was to build a real steam engine with alcohol as the fuel. I had been reading a magazine called *Steam in the Garden* and in it an article showed some of the steps involved in making a live steamer. A few books later and I was off in my workshop thinking about making the parts I saw in the books.

Along the way I meet some very helpful friends who gave me tips and encouragement to keep me going even when things did not work out. Two years later I had success and the Mogul, a 2-6-0 engine I was working on, ran! This first engine did not run very long, but it kept me going in the hobby.

One of the best things about the hobby is the friendships formed along the way. I now have friends around the world. About once a month we have get-togethers called steam-ups, and we go to each other's houses and run on the hoist tracks. Even our wives get into it and have a great time. It is a big social thing.

So far I have built about 15 live steam engines, some from kits and some from scratch. I find this a great way to relax in the evening after work. Machining small parts and planning are good mental exercise. At the end of the project, the reward is that I have made something, and with perseverance it can be made to run.

Profile and photo courtesy of Ernie Noa.

> *Implementation*

1. A variety of formats can be used, ranging from discussion initiated by participants to exploration of specified topics with a knowledgeable discussant. Each week's theme should be posted at least one week ahead.
2. Speakers from local universities or high schools, businesses, government offices, and organizations can provide both information and questions for discussion.

> *Options and Variations*

* Articles on the next week's topic can be posted online.
* Topics can vary from economics to philosophy (Kant, Foucault, Marx, Locke, Dewey, and so on) to social and other issues.
* Participants could plan and direct this program.

STARTING YOUR OWN BUSINESS

> *Description*

Having your own business has many advantages—and disadvantages. Find out what they are and how to get your business started. Participants will learn the components of writing a business plan, setting reasonable time lines, exploring funding options, and gaining access to supportive networks and resources.

> *Purpose and Goals*

* To learn the advantages and disadvantages of starting your own business
* To understand requirements and contents of a formal business plan
* To explore funding sources
* To establish a network for support

> *Length and Format*

A 3-hour workshop

> *Space*

Classroom

> *Staffing*

One instructor

> *Equipment and Materials*

* Tables and chairs
* Projection equipment (overhead transparency projector, PowerPoint projector, or both)
* Screen
* Handouts

> *Implementation*
>> 1. Present advantages and disadvantages of starting one's own business.
>> 2. Discuss creative, successful businesses as examples.
>> 3. Present the purpose and contents of each part of a business plan.
>> 4. Discuss sources of funding and the documentation needed for applying for funds.
>> 5. Provide a list of online and local organization networks and resources.

> *Options and Variations*
>> * Instructors may be recruited from the Small Business Administration (SBA), an organization of retired businesspeople, or current (successful) small business owners; or a banking executive or university professor could serve as instructor.
>> * A panel of small business owners may be invited to speak and also mingle with participants over refreshments.

TAKING THE MYSTERY OUT OF SUDOKU

> *Description*

Even Brad Pitt claims to be hooked on Sudoku. Ever wonder what the attraction is? Learn how to play this popular logic game.

> *Purpose and Goals*
>> * To understand the benefits of the logic game Sudoku
>> * To become familiar with forms of the game
>> * To learn how to play the game
>> * To exercise the brain by applying multiple techniques for solving the puzzles

> *Length*

One 2-hour workshop

> *Space*

Quiet room with tables and chairs; enough room for facilitator to move among the participants to give help

> *Staffing*

One teacher plus one staff per six to eight participants

> *Equipment and Materials*
>> * Large dry-erase board with Sudoku squares marked with colored masking or other tape
>> * Dry-erase markers
>> * Three different styles or levels of Sudoku puzzles (very easy, easy, and moderate) for each participant

* Pencil with a good eraser for each participant
* List of resources for more information
* Sample Sudoku puzzle books
* Sample Sudoku board

> *Implementation*

1. Provide background and history of Sudoku.
2. Show and explain the Sudoku grid layouts.
3. State the object and rules.
4. Demonstrate solution strategies.
5. Have participants try a simple puzzle, giving individual help when needed.
6. Explain more advanced strategies.
7. Provide help as participants try the next puzzle.
8. Provide a take-home Sudoku and review resources (where to find daily puzzles, books, boards).

> *Options and Variations*

* Can use overhead transparency with Sudoku grid marked or printed on it.
* Can use large paper with Sudoku grids; even the classified ads from newspapers will work with bright markers.

YOU AND YOUTUBE

> *Description*

Want to watch your grandchild's finals soccer game, or perhaps a comic episode from a movie? Learn how to use the Web media server YouTube, where anyone can post a video clip.

> *Purpose and Goals*

* To have a multimedia experience
* To acquire a knowledge base for a specific video Web site
* To learn ways to access this Web site and use it

> *Length and Format*

One 2-hour session

> *Space*

Large room with tables and chairs

> *Staffing*

One facilitator

➤ *Equipment and Materials*

* Hard copy of directions to hand out
* Large overhead screen
* Computers with Internet access—one hooked up to project onto screen

➤ *Implementation*

1. Show sample clips from YouTube.
2. Show the benefits of using this type of program and explain cautions.
3. Show participants how to access the Web site.

➤ *Options and Variations*

* Participants can work in pairs if the number of personal computers is limited.
* Have an additional, more advanced session in which participants can learn how to input their own video clips.

7

Life Is an Adventure

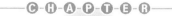

Outdoor Adventure Program Ideas

Rather than "activities," baby boomers enjoy *experiences.* Traveling "off the beaten path," waking up to a picturesque view of the mountains, riding a bike and feeling the wind swoosh past, or just enjoying a picnic with friends and a few ants may be attractive. Outdoor recreation offers a great variety of experiences, but the most sought after and increasingly popular is outdoor adventure; boomers are seeking a bit of risk in their outdoor experiences.

Boomers got their first taste of outdoor recreation in the 1950s and '60s when many boomers were children. Families purchased cars and began driving to visit outdoor areas, go camping, or have picnics. "Mobile homes" became popular as people traveled more. More and better roads were constructed to carry the increased traffic. Overall access to outdoor resources improved. Participation in outdoor recreation by all ages has increased steadily since that time, becoming more prominent and more active.

Outdoor recreation differs from other forms of recreation in its dependence on nature as a component of the activity. Snow is necessary for cross-country or downhill skiing, sledding, or snowboarding. Lakes, streams, and rivers provide places to fish, canoe, kayak, and run white-water rapids. Other natural features ensure our enjoyment of hiking, camping, leaf peeping, and bird watching. The interaction with nature inherent in these activities distinguishes them as outdoor recreation.

Outdoor recreation goes beyond the aesthetic surface and provides the participant with psychological, spiritual, and physical well-being benefits. In a study of 135 boomers, Cochran (2005) found that participation in outdoor leisure solely for the element of nature involved was favored by 63 percent of the men and 60 percent of the women. Seeking outdoor recreation for purposes of relaxation of mind, body, and spirit was noted by 42 percent of the men and 53 percent of the women. Participation in outdoor leisure for physical health or exercise was also important to 48 percent of the men and 45 percent of the women in the study. Boomers in general pursue outdoor leisure activities for relaxation, play, and continued growth.

According to the most recent National Sporting Goods Association survey (www.nsga.org), the most popular outdoor activities (i.e., those with the highest percentage of participation) for 45- to 54-year olds in the United States in 2007 included exercise walking, swimming, hiking, boating, golf, bicycle riding, and backpacking. Increasing in popularity were activities such as skateboarding, mountain biking, running and jogging, and fishing. These results were echoed in a study of active baby boomers and older adults conducted by Del Webb in 2007 (www.delwebb.com). The outdoor sports that this group (who live in communities designed for people aged 55 or older) ranked as extremely important were walking, swimming, golf, fishing, and canoeing/kayaking. Increasing in popularity were biking, hiking/climbing/rappelling, river rafting, downhill skiing, Rollerblading, competitive running, and hang gliding/parasailing/parachuting. It is clear that the boomers want to be physically active. One of the fastest-growing trends for this segment of the population is a form of outdoor recreation called adventure recreation. The key to making recreation "adventurous" is to add a calculated risk factor—some aspect of the activity that expands the participant's comfort zones. The risk may come from taxing one's physical skills, pushing one's mental capacities, or experiencing elements of danger.

Two factors are key for baby boomers who crave this type of recreation. First, when pushing one's limits, the risk must be calculated. For example, white-water rafting or rock climbing can be dangerous and deadly—even for seasoned participants. Baby boomers who are not experts need an experienced teacher or guide, good equipment, good safety gear, and instructions on what to do in case of a mishap. It is for this reason that we recommend contracting the professional services of experienced outfitters for adventure activities that have a moderate to high element of risk or danger. These outfitters should have trained leaders (be sure to check the outfitters' credentials) and should carry appropriate liability insurance (be sure to check their insurance).

Secondly, boomers like "soft" adventure. They are willing to work hard, get dirty and sweaty, and push their physical and mental limits. At the end of the day, however, they want a nice meal, perhaps with a glass of good wine, and a comfortable bed. The taste for soft adventure means that shorter trips and activities may be more attractive than longer ones.

MARKETING TIPS

When you are developing marketing campaigns for outdoor adventure programs, these are some important things to keep in mind:

- **You may not be objective.** As a programmer, you may love outdoor adventure activities. Because of your passion, you may have forgotten what it feels like to be a novice. But, to successfully market your programs to new customers, you must put yourself in your prospects' shoes, fins, hiking boots, skis, or flip-flops. You may not be objective enough to develop a marketing message that can effectively attract new participants. Promote the benefits of the program, not just the features. Be especially careful with jargon and slang. Many outdoor, extreme, and adventure activities involve a language and lingo all their own. Help customers feel comfortable in the outdoor recreation environment by avoiding words, phrases, and jargon that can make people feel like foreigners. No one wants to feel like an outsider—right, dude?

- **Safety sells.** Promote the safety of your programs. Adults, unlike children, understand that they are not invincible and may feel vulnerable when trying something new or risky. Stress the safety features and the safeguards associated with your program and equipment. Proudly showcase your staff's experience, education, awards, and certifications. While most children couldn't care less about your higher degrees in sport management, exercise physiology, or therapeutic recreation, many adults will be impressed and reassured by your credentials.

- **Flips might flop.** Don't depict the extreme side of a sport when trying to attract first-time participants. When designing ads, Web sites, and other marketing materials, try to show or otherwise include boomers (not teenagers or young adults) actually participating in the activity. Tony Hawk might be the perfect person to attract teenagers to skateboarding, but his thrills, chills, loops, and flips might scare the heck out of a baby boomer who is trying to get up the nerve to ride for the very first time.

- **Taste this.** Sampling is a great way to encourage people to try something new. Not only do samples eliminate financial risk since they are typically free, but they also appeal to our sense of curiosity. When it comes to outdoor recreation activities, look for ways for boomers to get a "taste" of an activity by offering free clinics, workshops, open houses, mini-sessions, or demos. While I might not want to invest a whole day in something new, like cross-country skiing, consider hosting an Adult Snow Day in which I can try several outdoor winter activities, including sledding, skiing, snowshoeing, snowmobiling, and ice fishing.

- **Cut expenses.** Outdoor recreation often requires expensive equipment. Help boomers wishing to try new activities to secure the equipment they need through some creative partnerships. For example, work with local retailers willing to loan or rent equipment or "demos" to program participants. Your agency might even invest in its own inventory of rental equipment, enabling first-timers to take part in outdoor recreation with little or no initial investment. As outdoor enthusiasts—young and old alike—become more advanced, they may be willing to donate or sell equipment to others. Your agency could sponsor (or cosponsor with your local sporting goods retailer) a community-wide gear-swap, helping to lessen recreation expenses.

OUTDOOR ADVENTURE PROGRAM IDEAS

The following activities serve as a guide to creating outdoor adventure programs with boomers. Adventure comes in many forms and does not have to involve actual high risk—only the *perception* of risk. Keep in mind that baby boomers tend to prefer smaller groups—which are also more appropriate than larger groups for adventure recreation. Be sure to include an educational component (e.g., learning how to put on your own climbing harness, learning how to "read" parts of the river) and a social component (perhaps as simple as a cup of coffee and a place to sit and chat with the activity group). Retelling of the adventure makes it memorable.

HIKING

> ### Description
> There is so much to see, discover, and learn during an adventure hike. Join us for a progressive hike on the Appalachian Trail. Enjoy a tasty, leisurely meal at the end.

> ### Purpose and Goals
> * To engage in a physical and cognitive activity
> * To socialize
> * To use problem-solving and leadership skills
> * To use various equipment and navigation tools

> ### Length and Format
> Half day or full day

> ### Space
> Well-marked hiking area

> ### Staffing
> One facilitator per six to eight participants, based on skill level of participants

> ### Equipment and Materials
> * Safety equipment (first aid kit, proper hiking attire)
> * Lunch for participants
> * Drinking water
> * Snacks
> * Navigation tools

> *Implementation*

1. Provide an orientation to the activity.
2. Review safety procedures.
3. Use a buddy system based on skill level.

> *Options and Variations*

* Any well-maintained hiking trail can be used.
* Adventure and trust-building activities can be added.
* Sensory experience activities can be added.
* Participants can plan the activity.

JET SKIING

> *Description*

Like the water? Planning a vacation in which motorized water sports will be available? Prepare by learning how to jet ski.

> *Purpose and Goals*

* To engage in a physical activity
* To acquire knowledge and skills to properly and safely use a motorized vehicle
* To apply new knowledge to a hands-on experience

> *Length and Format*

One 3-hour session

> *Space*

Outdoor setting with water

> *Staffing*

Depends on skill level

> *Equipment and Materials*

* Life jackets (personal flotation devices or PFDs)
* Water cones and buoys
* One jet ski per person
* Walkie-talkies

> *Implementation*

1. Use a dryland experience to teach parts of the machine, how to start and stop, proper riding technique, water travel etiquette, and safety.
2. Let participants apply the knowledge gained to use of the machine on water in a small area.
3. A group ride at the end of the session can be a culminating activity unless participants want to go off on their own.

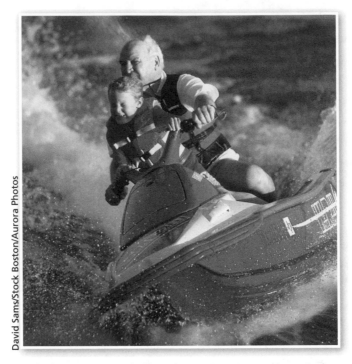

David Sams/Stock Boston/Aurora Photos

Baby boomers are thrill-seekers. Mature age doesn't slow them down!

> ### Options and Variations

    * Arrangements for participant discounts for additional rentals of equipment may be possible.

    * Start regular group rides as an ongoing leisure activity.

    * Participants may choose to partner up and ride together.

    * Races and obstacle courses can be set up for advanced riders.

    * A destination (island or nice picnic area along the shore) may be used.

TREASURE HUNTING: GEOCACHING AND GPS

> ### Description

Search for treasure as we learn to use global positioning system (GPS) to find a geocache (a site where current artifacts are buried). You will get to take the "treasure" home and leave your own for the next geocachers. Bring your hiking boots and an artifact (poem, drawing, small craft item, letter) to leave. Dress for the weather.

> ### Purpose and Goals

    * To learn to use GPS for guidance in the woods

    * To explore cross-country natural areas

* To socialize
* To connect with people you do not know

> *Length and Format*

One 2- to 3-hour session

> *Space*

Outdoor terrain with variety and interest

> *Staffing*

One leader and one staff member (in case of illness or accident)

> *Equipment and Materials*
  * GPS device
  * Maps
  * First aid kit
  * Drinking water
  * Clothing appropriate for weather conditions
  * Snacks

> *Implementation*
  1. Describe the purpose, history, and excitement of geocaching.
  2. Teach participants how to use the GPS device.
  3. Give safety instructions and guidelines for the adventure.

> *Options and Variations*
  * Before the trip, the leader should locate the site her- or himself so as to know the features of the terrain and cache site.
  * The Web site www.geocaching.com is a treasure trove in and of itself.

MOUNTAIN BIKING FOR WIMPS

> *Description*

Looking for an adventurous ride outside in the forest? Hop on a mountain bike and join us for an ultimate ride for anyone with any ability level.

> *Purpose and Goals*
  * To have an outdoor leisure experience
  * To have a social experience
  * To gain new knowledge and information you can use in the future in a recreation pursuit
  * To reach and achieve goals
  * To exercise the mind and body

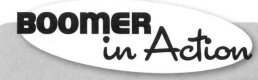

Sandy Johnson

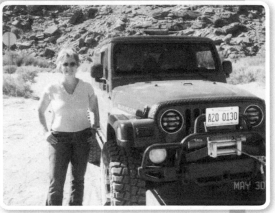

I remember when I was much younger, with three young children and a home in the country to care for, I saw a mud-covered "off-roader" driving down the street. At the time I wondered, "Why in the world would anyone want to do *that*?" But here I am, many years later, married to a man who is a born outdoor enthusiast, including what else—off-roading. He introduced me to his hobby in 1998, and we've been an off-roading couple ever since. The Jeep we use has been upgraded through the years, but taking the trails is still as exciting as it was the very first time in his MUTT (military utility tactical truck).

Each year we find ourselves loading up the trailer with our Jeep hitched to the Expedition and heading west to the Rockies. We've upgraded over time (another benefit of having older children), and we now are the proud owners of a red Jeep Rubicon. Last year we ventured into the beautiful red rock mountains of Moab, Utah, where we experienced a different kind of beauty and challenge. I love to drive the more moderate trails, and I let my husband handle those that are more difficult to traverse. The lure of the beautiful scenery of the mountains, as well as the challenge of negotiating the trails, is a hobby that I would not like to have missed in my journey here on this earth. I will admit that sometimes the trails get a bit frightful (such as Telluride's Black Bear), but I sure wouldn't want to trade the experience of seeing God's wonderful creations in this way.

Profile and photo courtesy of Sandy Johnson.

> *Length and Format*
> One 3-hour session

> *Space*
> Outdoor park and recreation area with cart paths or bike trails

> **Staffing**

One facilitator-leader

> **Equipment and Materials**

* Safety equipment (helmets, pads, first aid kit, repair kit)
* Mountain bikes with suspension

> **Implementation**

1. Give an overview of mountain biking.
2. Review parts of the bike and bike handling.
3. Teach techniques for easier riding.
4. Stress safety and trail etiquette.
5. Demonstrate use of a mountain bike.
6. Have participants practice techniques on a flat surface.
7. When participants are ready, take an easy group ride.

> **Options and Variations**

* Explain features to look for along the trail, history of the park, and so on.
* Provide information about mountain biking groups and trails.

CAMP GRANADA FOR GROWN-UPS

> **Description**

As you packed your kids off to camp, did you ever wish you could go back to camp yourself? Or, if you never went to camp before, here's your chance. You will go to Camp Granada, a camp for grown-ups who still have some kid inside! Swim in the lake. Raid the boys' or girls' cabin. Make s'mores, sing songs, and tell tall tales around the campfire.

> **Purpose and Goals**

To relive the camp experience in the great outdoors without Joe Spivey and his poison ivy

> **Length and Format**

About 1-1/2 days (arrive Saturday morning, leave Sunday after lunch)

> **Space**

Campground with bunkhouses, shower houses, waterfront, hiking trails

> **Staffing**

Ratio of one leader to 10 campers (including specialists such as canoe instructor, archery instructor, arts and crafts instructor). Don't forget the camp cook and camp nurse!

➤ *Equipment and Materials*

* Bedrolls or sleeping bags, brought by participants
* Food, food, and more food!
* Arts and crafts materials
* Sport equipment such as volleyball, canoes, archery equipment
* Instruments
* Campfire stories
* Gourmet s'mores (use small squares of dark [heart healthy] chocolate, mini-marshmallows, and graham crackers—a toned-down version of the original beast
* Acoustic guitars for camp songs, songs of the '60s, or whatever everyone knows the words to!
* Tambourines (can be made from dry rice, Dixie cups, a napkin, and a rubber band; or from paper plates and dry beans using a stapler)
* Comb instruments (small combs covered with tissue paper that is stretched tightly across the teeth of the comb—humming into the paper makes music)

➤ *Implementation*

1. Provide an orientation to camp, including risk management.
2. Include a typical camp itinerary with time for waterfront activities, arts and crafts, hiking, interactive games and contests (such as cabin decoration, silly Olympics, volleyball with a beach ball, initiative skills, hiking).
3. Have a camp song that staff teach campers during orientation. Sing it before meals, at the campfire, and at the close of the camp session.
4. Serve light, fresh, healthy (except for the s'mores) meals and snacks.
5. Be prepared for inclement weather by planning a lot of indoor games and activities.
6. Campers should have an official camp patch or pin or neckerchief to take home.

➤ *Options and Variations*

* Arrange a wine tasting without participants having to drive home.
* Have the participants decide the activities a few weeks before camp.

ADVENTURE TRAVEL: CANOEING

➤ *Description*

Do you enjoy the outdoors? Enjoy being on the water? Join us for a fantastic adventure in a canoe. Beginners, this one's for YOU!

> *Purpose and Goals*
  * To engage in an activity that addresses body, mind, and spirit
  * To have an opportunity for social interaction
  * To work with others as a team

> *Length and Format*
Half-day pretrip preparation and full-day trip

> *Space*
Large classroom for pretrip session plus swimming pool or lake or slow-moving river

> *Staffing*
One staff member per four to six students

> *Equipment and Materials*
  * Canoes (two or three participants per canoe)
  * One paddle per participant plus a couple of extras
  * Sunscreen
  * Dry clothes
  * Waterproof cushions
  * Food
  * Drinking water

> *Safety Equipment*
  * Well-fitted personal flotation devices (PFDs)
  * Water shoes
  * First aid kit

> *Implementation*
1. Have a dryland orientation to canoeing basics, safety procedures, the location, techniques, and what to bring to the activity. Assess the skill level of the participants. Orient the participants to the canoe and the additional equipment. Teach safety precautions (such as how to get in and get out of a canoe without tipping it over) and emergency techniques (what to do if the canoe overturns). Practice righting a canoe in the pool or in shallow water before the trip begins.
2. Guide the actual trip.
3. Take several breaks along the way, including stops for lunch in a nice spot and bathroom breaks.

> *Options and Variations*
  * Information about the environment would add interest.
  * Add fishing as an additional class.
  * Add a white-water river experience.

> Breathe. Let go. And remind
> yourself that this very moment is
> the only one you know you have
> for sure.
> —*Oprah Winfrey*

FLYING HIGH ABOVE 50 ADVENTURE CLUB

> ### Description

Up, up, and away . . . try your wings at forms of flight. Each month a different experience will be offered, from hot air balloons to parasailing to skydiving.

> ### Purpose and Goals

To have a safe and adrenaline-filled experience either to mark a milestone or just for the rush! This group can meet once a year, once a month, or more often as participants request.

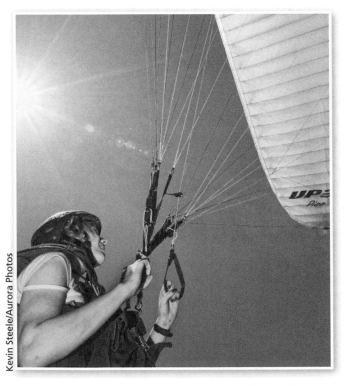

Kevin Steele/Aurora Photos

Paragliding is a sure way to get an adrenaline rush.

> *Length and Format*

Depend on activity and location. For example, hot air balloon rides may take a couple of hours, while skydiving requires on-the-ground teaching and preparation before the dive takes place.

> *Space*

Depends on activity

> *Staffing*

Contract with professionals who provide these experiences. Check out their credentials and insurance.

> *Equipment and Materials*

Transportation to the vendor (or participants meet at the site)

> *Implementation*

1. Contact local airport or flight school.
2. Group rates will be beneficial; look into pricing before establishing group sizes.

> *Options and Variations*

* Provide a T-shirt and photo opportunity. Contact your local newspaper for a media opportunity.
* Options might include hot air balloon rides, piloted ultralight or glider flights, tandem skydiving for a riskier adventure, or even bungee jumping.
* Tamer versions (but still adrenaline pumping) are the giant bungee trampolines that can be set up in a large parking area.

FOWL WEATHER FRIENDS: BIRD WATCHING SEMINAR AND EXCURSION

> *Description*

Tufted titmouse, slate gray junco, night hawk, wood thrush. . . . See and hear the common and the exotic birds that make up your neighborhood. Learn where and how to spot birds in their natural habitats. Learn their habits and where they live during the summer and winter. Identify their calls and songs.

> *Purpose and Goals*

* To learn new skills for spotting and identifying birds native to the area
* To exercise the senses

> *Length and Format*

A few hours to a weekend workshop

> *Space*

Outdoor area that attracts birds such as a park or open space bordered by woods

> *Staffing*

Knowledgeable birder as leader

> *Equipment and Materials*

* Extra binoculars for those who forget to bring theirs or do not have binoculars
* Bird identification field guides

> *Implementation*

1. This activity will take place over the course of two days. The first day is the seminar, and on the second day is a bird watching excursion. Participants should be asked to bring their own binoculars for the class. Provide a list of other gear (including information on dressing for the weather and in layers of clothing), water, food, snacks, and so on.
2. Hold a culminating experience with a day outing to a nearby state park; perhaps even arrive at the park before sunrise!

> *Options and Variations*

* You can provide transportation for the excursion or have participants meet at the excursion site.
* Provide lunch for participants (included in fee) or have them bring their own.
* You can conduct icebreakers throughout the day to encourage social interaction.
* You can provide a bird list to use as a check-off sheet as participants spot birds on the list.

NATURE SCAVENGER HUNT

> *Description*

Enjoy outdoor fun with your children and grandchildren. Meet in the park and join a good-natured (pun intended) scavenger hunt.

> *Purpose and Goals*

* To use teamwork to have a fun and exciting experience that raises the blood pressure in a good way
* To have intergenerational fun

> *Length and Format*

About 2 hours

> *Space*

Open field and nature trails

> *Staffing*

One staffperson per 25 participants

> *Equipment and Materials*
>   * Digital camera for each team
>   * Lists of items for teams to photograph
>   * Home base with viewing system for photos taken

> *Implementation*
>   1. Put together a list of objects found in nature (e.g., beech leaf, fern, spider web, worm casings, moss, mayflower, skunk cabbage, bird in a tree, squirrels, ants). Be creative! Assign point values (1-5) for each item.
>   2. Divide participants into teams (charge each person $5 so that you can have a prize for the winning team).
>   3. Set a time limit, and send everyone on their way.
>   4. Each team has a digital camera and is to take pictures of the items on the list; teams have to be back before the time limit runs out or are disqualified.
>   5. After everyone is back, view the pictures on a slide show and tally points. To make this more fun, make a laugh meter and give extra points to the team whose photos make the group laugh the most.

> *Options and Variations*
>   * Can be conducted in the city. Set up rules such that participants have to find everything in a specific city (e.g., library, pocket park, brownstone house, shoe store, grass growing out of a crack in the sidewalk, a dandelion, a ball field). To make the activity a little more challenging and fun, tell participants that they can't go to the mall.
>   * Participants can provide their own digital cameras or picture phones.

ADVENTURE TRAVEL: RAFTING FOR BEGINNERS

> *Description*
> A little adventure, a little action, a lot of fun! Shoot the rapids or drift along the current. Take part of a beginning-to-end journey down a white-water course.

> *Purpose and Goals*
>   * To engage in a physical activity
>   * To have a social experience
>   * To learn new skills

> *Length and Format*
> Half day and full day (pretrip meeting and trip)

> *Space*
>   * Large room for pretrip meeting
>   * Suitable river (water source)

> *Staffing*

One guide per four to six participants (best to contract these services)

> *Equipment and Materials*

Video with projection screen

> *Safety Equipment*

* Helmets
* Personal flotation devices (PFDs), properly fitted
* Wet suits if river is cold
* Water shoes
* Raft with paddles
* First aid gear
* Food
* Dry clothes
* Sunscreen
* Water

> *Implementation*

The trip should be guided for beginner levels. Provide an instructional video. Simulate motions and actions in the classroom and teach basic paddling techniques. Participants will be given specific safety training (how to safely pull someone who has fallen overboard back into the raft; how to orient oneself in the river if getting back into the raft is not an immediate option; what to do if the raft starts filling with water or gets stuck on a rock; what to do if the guide falls in, and so on). A stop will be made halfway through the trip to pull ashore for a lunch break.

> *Options and Variations*

* The guide will place one leader in charge. The trip is meant to be an enjoyable adventure, not a thrill-to-spill experience.
* Participants could take a nature walk or wade in a creek during the lunch break.
* A video or photos of the participants on their trip could be shown at a meeting a week or two after the trip.

QUADING

> *Description*

Try the latest off-road craze—quading. Learn how to start, drive, manipulate, have fun on, and stay safe on an all-terrain vehicle.

> *Purpose and Goals*

* To have an outdoor experience
* To try a new leisure activity

* To have the opportunity for a social experience
* To learn a popular motorized sport activity

> *Length and Format*

One 3-hour session

> *Space*

Large outdoor area that is not environmentally sensitive, with maneuverable obstacles

> *Staffing*

One facilitator (best to contract these services with reputable vendor)

> *Equipment and Materials*

All-terrain vehicles (ATVs)

> *Safety Equipment*

* Water to drink
* Sunscreen
* First aid equipment
* Helmet and other safety equipment as required by vendor

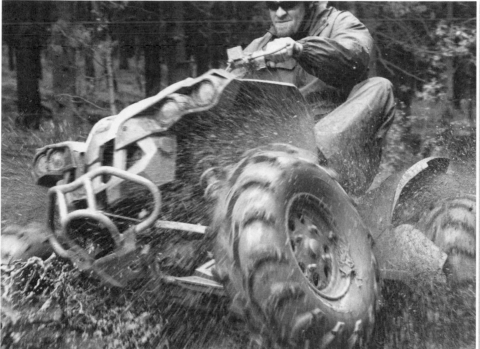

iStockphoto/Carrie Bottomley

Set up obstacle courses for all-terrain vehicles—and encourage boomers to get in there and get dirty!

> *Implementation*

1. Teach the parts of the vehicle.
2. Discuss precautions, safety features, and techniques, including how to minimize ecological damage.
3. Demonstrate how to start, ride, and stop safely.
4. Let participants enjoy a short outdoor ride.

> *Options and Variations*

* Participants can ride in pairs if they do not feel comfortable riding solo.
* You can set up a simple obstacle course to ride through.
* Additional social rides can be scheduled.
* Participants can join the local clubs for ATV riding (provide contact information).
* You can offer additional or advanced sessions if interest level is high.

PADDLE PADDLE KAYAK CLINIC

> *Description*

Kayaking gives you maneuverability to go where you want on the water. There are many different styles and types. This demonstration will feature how to find the right kayaks and paddles for the water you want to be on and for your body type and your strength. You get to try them out!

> *Purpose and Goals*

* To be introduced to safe, fun ways to kayak
* To learn how to select the proper boat and equipment

> *Length and Format*

Half day

> *Space*

Riverfront or lakefront

> *Staffing*

Depends on number of vendors and location. Be sure to include lifeguards in your staffing.

> *Equipment and Materials*

* A variety of kayaks
* A variety of paddles
* Personal flotation devices (PFDs)
* Dry bags and other gear for display (roof racks, seat pads, wet suits, and so on)

> *Implementation*

1. Contact a local canoe and kayak rental company or guide service to offer a partnership event that you will provide to participants with lots of

time and money to spend on recreation! The vendor sets up the facility and the boats and provides certified instructors; make sure to visit the facility before offering partnership, and make sure it's a clean and safe place to have fun.

2. Demonstrate the actions of different paddles, paddling techniques, dryland boat features, on-the-water boat handling, and equipment.

3. You could also hold mini-clinics on finding the right PFD, selecting a paddle, improving paddling techniques, paddling for beginners, rolling the boat, and so on.

4. Time on the water for participants to try out the equipment is a must.

> ### Options and Variations
This program could be held at a river or lake or at the ocean.

TANDEM KAYAKING

> ### Description
Enjoy kayaking through creeks and down rivers with a companion or guide in your boat. Tandem kayaking allows for two people to have their own seat in the same boat. Enjoy the trip together.

> ### Purpose and Goals
* To improve physical strength
* To increase communication and cooperation
* To enjoy the outdoors

> ### Length and Format
One hour, half day, full day

> ### Space
Outdoor area with waterfront

> ### Staffing
Depends on participants' experience

> ### Equipment and Materials
* Tandem kayaks, one for every two participants
* Personal flotation devices (PFDs)
* Safety information
* Paddles
* First aid kit
* Drinking water
* Snacks
* Sunscreen
* Field guides

➤ *Implementation*

Introduce participants to water safety and boating guidelines. Have participants sit in kayaks on land and practice maneuvers, strokes, communication,
and other pertinent techniques they may be using when in the water. Have
participants take boats to the water and do some skills and drills sessions.
Take group on a guided tour.

➤ *Options and Variations*

* Participants can stop to look at interesting natural features.
* You can plan relay races and competitions during the day.

8

Move to the Beat

● ● ● ● ● ● ● ● ● ● ● ● ●

Healthy Living Program Ideas

Sport, fitness, and wellness activities are essential to good health and well-being. The benefits of physical activity are well publicized: increased cardiovascular health and reduced severity or delay of onset of diseases such as diabetes, Alzheimer's, and osteoporosis. The effectiveness of exercise in mitigating the effects of stress and depression is also well documented.

An obsession with fitness is one of the main identifying characteristics of the boomer generation. As you have read in earlier chapters, baby boomers in general seem intent on feeling young, being healthier, and living longer. Thus as a group, boomers have a determined mind-set, do not recognize limits, and are not allowing the aging process to affect their lives negatively (Bales, 2001). Boomers believe they will live longer than prior generations and are already implementing healthier lifestyles in their retirement, for example, through exercise and positive eating habits.

Despite the emphasis on fitness, only 26 percent of boomers exercise regularly, 20 percent exercise infrequently, and a whopping 53 percent do not bother to exercise at all (Thornhill & Martin, 2007). But the importance of becoming or staying physically active is clear.

Some baby boomers enjoy competition. Activities such as Senior Olympics and masters sports support the desire for competition in age-appropriate contexts and venues. For those who are not so competition oriented, enjoyment is the key to starting and maintaining regular physical activity. Support is essential to sustaining the motivation to remain engaged. A powerful connection exists between social connections and continued success in exercise and weight loss programs (McGonigal, 2007).

With regard to recreation activities and retirement, some boomers have the same interests as the generation before them; however, most boomers desire more active forms of lifestyle programming. In a comparative study of boomers and recreation professionals (Cochran, 2005), both groups identified the recreation activities that they thought boomers participated in at the time and the activities they thought boomers would participate in during their retirement. There were two especially noticeable differences. First, boomers said that movies, camping, and sewing were among their top 10 activities, whereas recreation professionals thought that boomers' top activities included taking university courses and learning about investments and finance. Secondly, boomers listed activities that might be considered unusual and that recreation professionals had not listed, such as learning to surf, paragliding, running a marathon, skydiving, river running, bungee jumping, hang gliding, riding ATVs, wine making, climbing, owning a business, learning a new language, and learning how to play a musical instrument. Clearly the boomer expectations indicate a healthy, vibrant lifestyle.

As leaders of America's health revolution, boomers are physically capable of working and producing much later in life than any previous generation simply because they have taken care of themselves and will continue self-care into the next phase of their lives. Also note that personal well-being in boomers is enhanced through their leisure rather than by monetary income (Cochran, 2005). Again, boomers expect to live an active, healthy lifestyle.

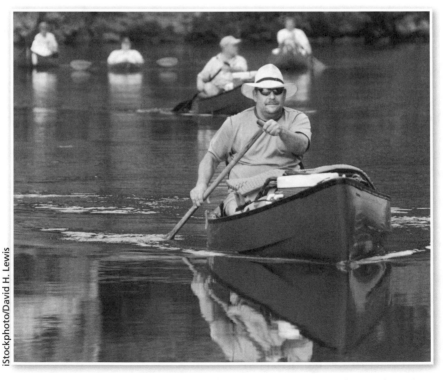

iStockphoto/David H. Lewis

Canoeing is a great way to get exercise, explore nature, and socialize all at the same time.

As we have already noted, boomers plan to carry their willingness to learn new things, their desire for challenge, and their passion for education and culture with them into retirement and into their recreation activity interests. You should take all of these components into consideration when you are developing programs for this unique cohort. From a programming perspective, "We may anticipate the growing demands for recreational resources which are utilized by physically fit, health-conscious consumers who happen to be of retirement age" (Todd, 2004).

MARKETING THAT MOVES PEOPLE TO ACTION

There's probably not a boomer alive who doesn't know that active living and exercise are good for the body, mind, and soul. But that doesn't mean that everyone is ready to get up off the couch and get moving. Getting boomers to embrace or reembrace fitness and sport programs will involve challenges directly associated with their age and stage in life—as well as some good old-fashioned pride. For example, those who participated in sports as children, teenagers, or young adults might feel frustrated by their lack of agility, flexibility, balance, or stamina. Rather than ignore this frustration, acknowledge it in marketing materials.

Others, especially women, may feel anxious and self-conscious about donning a swimsuit or form-fitting active wear in front of complete strangers. If you have private dressing rooms or women's-only workout areas, make sure to promote these features loud and clear to female boomers. In general, when marketing fitness programs to baby boomers, keep the "steps to the buy" (chapter 3) close at hand. Pay particular attention to initial motivators such as vanity and emerging health concerns as you develop your marketing message.

It is also important for you and your younger staff to avoid judging boomers based on their current physical condition. Today's out-of-shape baby boomer may have been yesteryear's high school football hero, track star, or award-winning swimmer. Train staff to be compassionate, considerate, and respectful of boomers no matter what their size, shape, or skills. Your ability to kindly walk a boomer through those critical first steps of an unfamiliar activity may make the difference between repelling a new customer and developing a lifelong love of a game.

Once again, remember to augment marketing efforts by collaborating with other fitness centers, health clubs, and sport programs. Together you can ensure the perfect mix and variety of fitness programs for every boomer in your service area, from former Olympian to first-timer.

When choosing graphics for fitness programs aimed at boomers, create ads using photos of healthy, happy-looking men and women who are approximately 15 years younger than your target audience. The skewed self-image of boomers requires marketers to carefully select a younger role model (but not too much younger) to attract today's older adult.

Fitness programs can meet the needs of participants, volunteers, and fans alike. With this in mind, work to build relationships with your active customers that involve more than their physical abilities to swing, kick, or throw. This is especially important when you are dealing with aging boomers. As people age, most experience physical and emotional conditions that may impede, limit, or—sadly—end their ability to participate in activities they once loved. Rather than lose good customers to ailments, disabilities, or illness, look for other less strenuous ways to keep them connected to your program.

For example, you may have an avid tennis player who begins suffering from arthritis, making it painful and eventually impossible to hold a racket. However, that player might make a fantastic coach for a youth team. Or perhaps he or she could participate in tournaments as scorekeeper, line judge, or volunteer. Recreation programs may not offer the physical benefits they once did; but they can still provide critical social benefits, reducing alienation, depression, loneliness, and other maladies often associated with the aging process.

HEALTHY LIVING PROGRAM IDEAS

Physical activity is essential to physical and emotional functioning and to the healthy functioning of the brain. The following program ideas will help you and your movers move to the beat. Programs include dance, exercise, and fitness and have to do with generally taking care of oneself.

MORE THAN JUST A WALK IN THE PARK

> *Description*

A day of low-, moderate-, and high-energy activities—all designed to make you healthier. Find the ones that fit you best and learn where to access these activities in the community.

> *Purpose and Goals*

To experience a day of education, social recreation, and awareness of physical health

> *Length and Format*

Half day

> *Space*

Large room with space for exhibits and demonstrations or open field or park area

> *Staffing*

* Staff to give directions and help with setup
* Supervisory staff for each "event"

> *Equipment and Materials*
  * Directional signs (events, rest rooms, parking, and so on)
  * Program brochure with map of exhibits and location of events

> *Implementation*
  1. Ideas for stations include chair exercises, seated massage, healthy snacks, blood pressure and cholesterol screenings, healthy cooking, tai chi, balance ball, hula hoop, and other fitness class demonstrations (Dance Revolution, Zumba, salsa dancing, Pilates, and so on).
  2. Events could include demonstrations, 5K walk, 10K run, dog walk, nature hike.

> *Options and Variations*
  * Local businesses can provide services, giveaways, coupons, and so on.
  * You can also coordinate with hospitals and gyms.
  * This could be an intergenerational event with active games (old-fashioned sack races, clothes relays, Whiffle ball games, and so on).

VIRTUAL GUITAR

> *Description*

This is your chance to be in that rock band, the way you always wanted! Use the television and game system to play the guitar—you do not need to know how to play. The game will do it for you.

> *Purpose and Goals*
  * To have an interactive experience
  * To have a musical experience
  * To exercise cognitive and motor skills

> *Length and Format*

Any length and format

> *Space*

Enough space for players to have an arm's length between them

> *Staffing*

One person to set up the equipment; participants will self-direct

> *Equipment and Materials*
  * Playstation 2 or 3 system
  * Television
  * Guitar Hero (instrument)

> ### Implementation

Connect gaming system and turn television on. Participants follow instructions on the screen to choose a character, song, instrument, and level of play. Instructional demos, practice songs, and helpful hints are provided. Colored keys on the system guitar allow the participant to play along with the song being projected on the television. By pressing the corresponding color key as it falls to the bottom of the TV screen, the participant stays synchronized with the rocker on the screen.

> ### Options and Variations

* Rock band: Have participants create their own groups—several people can play at the same time.
* Competitions can be held.

GALACTIC BOWLING BLAST

> ### Description

Black lights, disco music, bowling balls, and pins that glow in the dark! Join the fun for this galactic gala.

> ### Purpose and Goals

* To socialize with peers
* To get some exercise in a unique way

> ### Length and Format

Two-hour session

> ### Space

Bowling alley that offers glow-in-the-dark bowling (bowling alleys can often reserve times, days, or nights for special groups)

> ### Staffing

One staffperson for on-site registration

> ### Equipment and Materials

Provided by the bowling alley

> ### Implementation

Participants must preregister.

> ### Options and Variations

Transportation can be provided by your agency, or participants can arrive on their own. Glow-in-the-dark necklaces and bracelets add charm. Many different configurations can add interest: male teams versus female teams, mixed-gender and mixed skill-level teams (for example, set a maximum total handicap for any given team), novices-only night, birthday bowling).

CHEERLEADING SQUAD

> *Description*

Get out your tennis shoes and dust off your pom-poms. Join the cheerleading squad. No prior experience necessary, but you must be willing to learn, have a good time, and shake that booty—all in good taste! We will prepare to perform at the Senior Games.

> *Purpose and Goals*

* To be physically active while having fun
* To be mentally active by learning new moves

> *Length and Format*

Three 2-hour clinics followed by weekly practices during the six months prior to the Games

> *Space*

Large room with wooden floor

> *Staffing*

Coach-choreographer (university students who have coached cheerleading and dance majors may make suitable coaches)

> *Equipment and Materials*

* Uniforms and equipment such as pom-poms (to be provided by participants)
* Sound equipment for music, such as a boom box

> *Implementation*

1. Cheerleading clinics should be held first to teach the fundamentals and safety. Then choreography can be taught and practiced in subsequent sessions.
2. Tryouts for the final squad can be held.
3. If participants want to get competitive, a national contest is held at the National Senior Olympic Games.

> *Options and Variations*

* Participants should be required to provide a doctor's note stating that they can participate.
* Avoid jumping moves—stick to dance steps to music and verbal cheers.
* Performance can take place during basketball half-time or community events.
* Fund-raising can be done to purchase uniforms.

JOIN THE DANCE REVOLUTION

> *Description*

Learn the latest dance steps—quickly and easily, at your own pace. Join others to follow the prompts for placing your feet for dance steps. Lots of fun!

> *Purpose and Goals*

* To get an aerobic workout
* To have fun with other people

> *Length and Format*

May be best as a drop-in

> *Space*

Open fitness room or gym

> *Staffing*

Staff to do the hookup (once it is in place, typed directions can be posted and participants can go at their own pace)

> *Equipment and Materials*

Nintendo Wii platform, cords, and dance pads

> *Implementation*

This activity can be led or supervised by a staffperson, or directions can be posted near the equipment. The activity is best if done in small social groups.

> *Options and Variations*

* Pace, music, and difficulty of steps can be varied.
* You may follow (or begin) the activity with an instructor-led class or clinic.

QUINTATHLON

> *Description*

If you enjoy team competition, with each team member having her or his own expertise, then you'll enjoy the challenge of the quintathlon. Instead of the usual running, biking, and swimming of a triathlon, this race will include FIVE-member teams and FIVE event segments: walking, biking, canoeing, swimming, and kayaking.

> *Purpose and Goals*

* To physically challenge yourself
* To exercise in a competitive atmosphere
* To work with others as a team

> *Length and Format*

One-time event

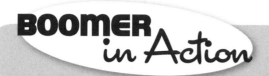

BOOMER in Action

Jan Kiehl

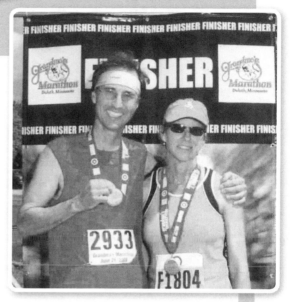

I've always been active. Even though I'm 54, my level of activity hasn't changed all that much, although the intensity certainly has. My primary activity is running, something my husband and I do together (he's also 54). We've been lucky that our race paces are similar so that we can be training partners, which has helped us keep at it for more than 25 years. We now run five days a week instead of six, we don't do any two-a-days like we did in our 30s, and the speed work is less intense than it used to be. We typically run 35 to 45 miles per week, depending on what we're training for; we also walk the dogs 3 miles twice a week.

We still do quite a few races each year. My favorite distance is the half-marathon. We recently ran Grandma's Marathon in Duluth, Minnesota, and qualified for Boston, which we plan to run in April 2009.

By profession I am the recreation manager for the City of Thornton, Colorado, so I am very lucky in that my job is all about recreation and my office is in a recreation center. So in addition to my running, I try to cross-train two or three lunch hours per week, typically doing various types of cardio (elliptical, arc trainer, step mill, and treadmill).

At home, we have a great workout room and my husband and I do our strength training in the evenings. This is the area where I need to be more disciplined. I need to lift weights two or three times per week, but we struggle to stay consistent. I also typically do additional cardio at home on the weekend (elliptical, arc trainer, and treadmill). I have dabbled with reformer Pilates and really enjoyed it, but I struggle to get to the studio, which isn't as handy as my basement.

Profile and photo courtesy of Jan Kiehl.

➤ *Space*

A park with river or lake and separate trails for biking and walking

➤ *Staffing*

Overall competition director, registration staff, event segment coordinators or supervisors, judges, first aid personnel, timers, direction givers and equipment staff, and concessions to sell items such as bottled water and healthy snacks

➤ *Equipment and Materials*

* Printed numbers with safety pins for competitors
* Scorecards and pencils
* Registration materials and waivers
* Timing devices
* First aid materials
* Starting line markers
* Loud starting device (such as whistle or air horn)
* Finish line tape
* Prizes
* Directional signs

➤ *Implementation*

This is a great event for involving volunteers or raising money for a cause. Volunteers must be trained in safety, emergency procedures, and other tasks such as timing competitors.

➤ *Options and Variations*

Activities such as biking, running, and canoeing are traditionally popular in triathlons. Different types of activities can be included. For children and more spontaneous adults, activities that are more fun and whimsical, such as river tubing, may be included. Activities such as tandem kayaking or team rowing could allow persons with disabilities to participate.

WHIFFLE BALL DERBY

➤ *Description*

Take me out to the (Whiffle) ball game. The smell of the hot dogs, popcorn, and peanuts . . . the cheer of the crowd . . . the crack of the bat—well, maybe more like a thunk of the bat because it's plastic, and so is the ball. Come out to the ballpark for the Whiffle Ball Derby. No prior experience needed; it's all fun!

> *Purpose and Goals*
>
> * To exercise large muscles
> * To socialize

> *Length and Format*

Two hours for one or more games

> *Space*

Softball field (depending on age and fitness level of participants, boundaries can be moved closer to home plate)

> *Staffing*

* Supervisory staff
* Umpire
* Coaches to be chosen by teams

> *Equipment and Materials*

* Whiffle balls
* Whiffle bats
* Bases

> *Implementation*

1. Use the same rules as softball—or change them!
2. Have players sign a code of conduct.

> *Options and Variations*

* You can allow more strikes, or batters can bat until they hit the ball.
* High school booster teams can run the concession stand.
* You can mix males and females on the same team, but try to balance the number of each sex across all teams.
* Novice nights allow people with low or no skills to play without feeling out of place.
* You can use middle school, high school, or park and recreation fields.
* You can have participants play without teams—they simply rotate positions (as in volleyball) as each new batter comes to bat.
* Rather than pitting one team against the other, you can keep a cumulative score.

Just play. Have fun. Enjoy the game.
—*Michael Jordan*

NINTENDO WII SPORTS

> **Description**

Beat your friends at sports—even if you've never played before. Nintendo Wii allows you to simulate a variety of sports including tennis, bowling, and soccer without hurting your knees or back. Bring a friend and play informally or join a league.

> **Purpose and Goals**

* To maintain hand–eye coordination and exercise the brain
* To get moderate arm exercise
* To socialize with others

> **Length and Format**

One-hour sessions with teams

> **Space**

About 10 by 10 feet, clear of obstacles

> **Staffing**

If directions are posted, no staffing needed except to boot up the software

> **Equipment and Materials**

Nintendo game station and accessories; television

> **Implementation**

Enlarge and post the directions that come with the games.

> **Options and Variations**

* This works best with a small social group.
* A league can be set up and scores posted.
* Teams can play at their own convenient times without the opposing team present.
* High scorers can be posted.

WINTER MINI-TRIATHLON

> **Description**

Sample fun triathlon events before taking on a bigger challenge. Three-person teams are needed to compete—form your own, or we'll find a team for you. Cross-country ski, snowshoe, and propel a hockey sled across the pond for a sense of accomplishment and light competition.

> **Purpose and Goals**

* To get physical exercise outdoors
* To socialize with others
* To "test the waters" with sport competition

> *Length and Format*

One-time event (or two times a season)

> *Space*

Outdoor space with snow and varied terrain—a city park, state park, or golf course may suffice

> *Staffing*

A great event to involve volunteers in—requires overall competition director; registration staff; event coordinators and judges; first aid personnel; direction givers and equipment staff; and concessions to sell items such as coffee, hot chocolate, bottled water, and healthy snacks

> *Equipment and Materials*

  * Large numbers with safety pins for competitors
  * Scorecards and pencils
  * Registration materials and waivers
  * Timing devices
  * First aid materials

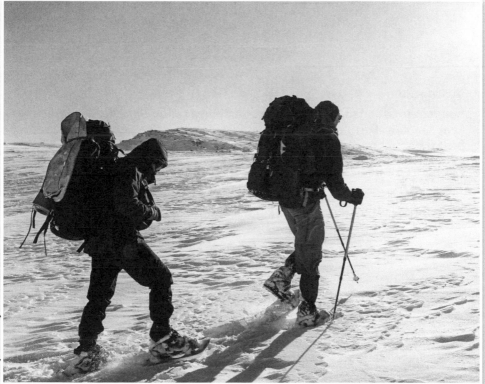

iStockphoto/Galyna Andrushko

Snowshoeing is one of many ways to get out and enjoy the winter wonderland. Be sure to have hot cocoa ready when they come back!

* Starting line markers
* Loud starting device (such as whistle or air horn)
* Finish line tape
* Prizes
* Directional signs

> **Implementation**

1. This is a great event for involving volunteers or raising money for a cause. Volunteers must be trained in safety, emergency procedures, and other tasks such as timing competitors.
2. If the number is large, the entrants can be divided into three groups, each starting at a different event.

> **Options and Variations**

Activities such as downhill skiing and snowshoeing are traditionally popular. Different types of activities can be included. For children and more spontaneous adults, activities that are more whimsical and fun such as tubing down a hill, snow person building, snowball contests (toss for distance, toss for accuracy), or snow sculpturing can be used. Activities such as moving sledge hockey sleds across a pond or tethered skiing (sit ski attached to cross-country skier with a tether) could allow persons with disabilities to participate.

YOGALATES

> **Description**

Reduce stress and increase balance, flexibility, range of motion, and strength. Feel calm. Feel great! Yogalates combines the best of yoga and Pilates for a great whole-body and mind workout.

> **Purpose and Goals**

* To reduce stress
* To increase flexibility and range of motion
* To improve balance
* To increase strength

> **Length and Format**

One to three classes per week, 1 hour each

> **Space**

A quiet room with controlled temperature, large enough for all participants to lie down a minimum of one arm's length apart

> **Staffing**

Certified instructor

➤ *Equipment and Materials*
  * Equipment—can be brought by participants; for those who do not have their own, one of the following for each person:
    • Mat
    • Blanket
    • Pilates block
    • Pilates-type strap
  * Sound equipment such as CD player or iPod amplifier

➤ *Implementation*

Utilize the services of a certified instructor who has a good reputation in the community. The instructor will design the classes and sequence of activities.

➤ *Options and Variations*

Everyone has a different body rhythm. Scheduling classes at several different times of the day will accommodate the varying needs.

TAKE CHARGE OF YOUR BODY

➤ *Description*

Get fit and eat well the easy way. This program will help you understand when, why, and how to exercise. You will also learn what and how to eat to stay healthy. You will develop strategies for your own personalized wellness program that is manageable and easy to follow.

➤ *Purpose and Goals*
  * To develop a program geared to individual needs for healthy eating
  * To develop a program that meets individual needs for fitness exercise
  * To develop workable methods for measuring success
  * To develop individual strategies for adhering to the wellness plan

➤ *Length and Format*

Two 10-week classes, about 1-1/2 hours each (potential topics listed under "Implementation")

➤ *Space*

Meeting room

➤ *Staffing*

One facilitator for each topic area

➤ *Equipment and Materials*
  * Table
  * Chairs
  * Audiovisual equipment
  * Handouts
  * Samples of exercise bands and balls

> *Implementation*

Each class should have a different focus and should be led by a community expert in that area. Potential topics include why exercise (benefits), exercise and the brain, assessing body mass index (BMI), goal setting, understanding nutrition labels, new Food and Drug Administration (FDA) guidelines for nutrition, sampler of "diet" books (pros and cons), the importance of stretching, building daily support, how to get back on track when you slip off, getting motivated, staying motivated, building a buddy system, measuring success, using exercise bands, using balance balls safely, handling sore muscles, eating out healthily, how to be more conscious of what you eat, identifying events that trigger impulse eating, simple exercises for anywhere and any time, and others geared specifically to the participants' needs.

> *Options and Variations*

  * Sources of experts for nutrition: local hospital dietician, private nutrition specialists, university professors

  * Sources of experts for exercise: YMCA fitness staff, exercise physiology instructors or graduate students, fitness center staff

  * Sources of experts on motivation and strategies: counselors, social workers, motivational speakers, people who have succeeded in their own wellness programs

  * Other resources: local bookstore, Weight Watchers, doctors who specialize in weight issues, sport clinic staff

ALTERNATIVE THERAPIES HEALTH FAIR

> *Description*

Oh, those little aches and pains. At this event you will learn how to treat them without adding more chemicals to your body.

> *Purpose and Goals*

  * To be introduced to nonintrusive methods of treatment
  * To find out about community resources for alternative therapies
  * To expand options for health care

> *Length and Format*

Open-house format, about 3 to 4 hours

> *Space*

Large space with good foot traffic circulation, good parking needed for people who come and go

> *Staffing*

On-site event manager plus staff to troubleshoot; extra staff for setup and takedown

> *Equipment and Materials*
  * Directional signs
  * Table and a chair for each exhibitor; trash cans

> *Implementation*
  1. In contract notes for exhibitors, make them responsible for setup and cleanup of their own space. Setup should be complete at least 1/2 hour before the event opens to the public. Exhibitors need to stay until the event is closed to the public and should be finished cleaning up within 1/2 hour.
  2. Also note in writing that business cards and brochures may be distributed but that on-site selling cannot take place.
  3. Suggestions to include:
     * Massage
     * Bone density
     * Arthritis prevention
     * Aromatherapy
     * Acupuncture
     * Reiki
     * Cosmeceuticals

> *Options and Variations*
  * This would be a good collaborative event with the local hospital.
  * Demonstrations may be included.

ZUMBA

> *Description*

Shimmy off those excess pounds. This dance-aerobics workout is for all ages. Fantastic Latin music, footwork that we'll teach you step by step, and lots of fun.

> *Purpose and Goals*
  * To improve physical fitness
  * To improve balance
  * To improve coordination

> *Length and Format*

One hour, three times a week for six to eight weeks

> *Space*

Large space without obstacles; chairs off to the sides; preferably mirrors lining one wall (as in a dance studio)

> **Staffing**

Trained instructor

> **Equipment and Materials**

* Printed handouts of directions for steps
* Sound system
* Good Latin music (usually furnished by instructor)
* Microphone for instructor

> **Implementation**

Instructions for clothing and footgear need to be given ahead of time.

> **Options and Variations**

* Participants must have permission of their doctor to participate in aerobic activity.
* Participants with balance issues may want to hold on to a chair while doing the steps.

9

Hit the Road

Travel Program Ideas

Ever since ancient times, people have traveled for pleasure. Travel is one of the trends in baby boomer leisure pursuits. From small day trips to extended tours, this generation seeks experiences that are informative and educational. It is interesting to note that when asked if they planned to travel more than their peers, African Americans and Hispanics/Latinos said yes nearly twice as often as white non-Hispanics (Thornhill & Martin, 2007).

Four areas of travel emerge as having high interest among the boomers: intergenerational, service, culture and heritage, and "field-to-plate." Each of these areas provides the key elements of education and adventure. Keep in mind that this kind of travel must also include amenities and comfort.

Instead of using the program planning format as in earlier chapters of the book, this chapter provides several examples of each trend. We recommend using trained experts to arrange trips and tours. Travel companies will often provide free spots on tours for your agency staff when a minimum number of participants have paid.

INTERGENERATIONAL TRAVEL

Half of all grandparents in the United States are baby boomers (Thornhill & Martin, 2007). In keeping with the boomers' desire to recreate with family and in small, intimate groups, some travel companies and destination sites specialize in intergenerational travel.

According to the Travel Industry Association of America (TIA), a full 30 percent of traveling grandmothers have taken at least one trip with a grandchild. Even more surprising were the results of a study by industry

> **Our heritage and ideals, our code and standards—the things we live by and teach our children—are preserved or diminished by how freely we exchange ideas and feelings.**
> —*Walt Disney*

consultants Yesawich, Pepperdine, Brown and Russell, which showed that almost 60 percent of kids ages 6 through 17 would really like to vacation with their grandparents.

Day trips involve special local and regional events and activities such as pumpkin festivals; apple picking; sugar bush tours, followed by pancakes with maple syrup, of course; specialized farming such as alpaca or emu farms; and cultural festivals.

Longer trips include destinations of interest to all ages. On a tour, participants may get to walk through the ruins of cities 10,000 years old, observe wildlife in their natural habitat, look at the night lighting on past American presidents' faces carved into a huge cliff side, and see mud pots boil and Old Faithful erupt.

The travel companies that specialize in intergenerational travel include GrandTravel (www.grandtrvl.com) and Generations Touring Company (www.generationstouringcompany.com). GrandTravel offers trips exclusively for grandparents and their grandchildren. The GrandTravel Web site provides a brief history of the beginnings of the business:

> Developed by a team of teachers, psychologists, and leisure counselors, GrandTravel is dedicated to helping grandparents create lasting memories for themselves and their grandchildren. (www.grandtrvl.com, Home page)

Trips for 2008 have Alaska as a destination with the promise of "glaciers, gold mines, and salmon fishing." River rafting, wildlife viewing at Denali National Park, a tour in a helicopter that lands on a glacier, and a visit to a dogsled camp—followed by a ride on a dogsled across a glacier—are some of the attractions that help make those lasting memories.

The Trains of the Old West tour includes history, Native American and Mexican culture, and visits to a national monument, a national park, and a World Heritage site (Taos Pueblo). Aztec dancers, a Diné (Navajo) storyteller, and artists share glimpses into their cultures. Exploring old mining towns and a ghost town sparks tales and imagination. The featured steam engine train rides offer scenic views and a look at the era when trains were vital to the economy.

In addition, many travel companies offer special family packages. Even Elderhostel (www.Elderhostel.com) and Smithsonian Journeys offer intergenerational trips. Destinations are national and international: Alaska wilderness coastline, Native American Southwest, New Zealand, Greece, Tanzania, Galapagos Islands. Smithsonian "family programs" feature this opportunity:

> Kayak, snorkel, and hike the shores and waters of the archipelago to witness unique animal behavior and habitats. Visit the Charles Darwin Research Center to learn about the ongoing and vital preservation work that is conducted by the Center. (www.darwinfoundation.org, Home page)

Destination sites also provide intergenerational programming. For example, the Great Camp Sagamore Historic Site in upstate New York offers a special long weekend for grandparents and grandchildren. Participants stay in a rustic yet comfortable lodge; meals are family style. The program includes separate activities for the "grans" and the grandchildren. The grandchildren may expend their energy and excitement with trained staff in the woods by learning how to "read" the presence of wildlife, making twine from native plants, or hiking up a nearby "mountain." Meanwhile, the grandparents can

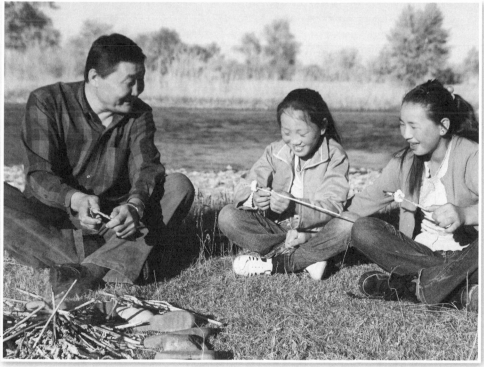

iStockphoto/Robert Churchill

Reinforce the importance of family by offering multigenerational activities, such as camping.

simply relax, listen to folklore as recounted by a skilled storyteller, or make their own wooden canoe paddle. Joint activities might include learning how to canoe, making baskets, taking nature walks, and singing around a campfire at night—complete with s'mores.

SERVICE TRAVEL

Baby boomers volunteer more than any other age cohort. Moreover, nearly half have said that they intend to volunteer more during retirement. The combination of travel and service becomes very attractive for many. And, yes, boomers are willing to pay to go to another country or another part of the United States in order to work. The key is that the work must be meaningful, products must be visible, and hardships must be minimized.

Boomers are traveling to places such as Guatemala, Malawi, and Kuwait to help harvest crops, paint schools, teach English, build water systems, tend infants and toddlers in orphanages, build churches, teach basic health skills, assist with clinics, and teach food preservation skills. At some destinations, the service workers are housed and fed in local homes. In others, housing is in a hotel or university dormitory. In all locations, opportunities to interact with local people and take photos that document the experience are essential, as are a comfortable and safe place to sleep and enough food and water.

Essential for agency program staff is a reputable source to plan and lead these trips. Professional association list servers are often a good source. These allow you to send a query to learn from others whom they recommend and why. Be sure to check the Better Business Bureau and to find out about the cancellation rate from the agency providing the services.

CULTURE AND HERITAGE TRAVEL

The rise in interest in genealogy is indicative of many boomers seeking reconnections, or even first connections, with family roots. Travel to places of origin of their families is a growing trend. While providing trips to each individual's ancestral hometown is impossible, many boomers are satisfied with gaining a flavor of their country of origin. Observation alone will not satisfy. Taking a simple tour of a quaint vineyard in Tuscany, attending a harvest dance in a Kenyan village, or observing a tea ceremony in Tokyo is not enough. The entire trip must provide education about and interaction with the culture and people. At a tea ceremony, for example, visitors may dress in kimonos; hear about the tying of the obi; learn about kinds of teas and how to select the different kinds; get explanations of the service itself— the meaning, symbolism, and ritual; and actually perform some part of the ceremony. A visit to the vineyard might include an explanation of why certain kinds of grapes can grow in particular microclimates, how the soil affects the taste of the grape, and how workers know when the grapes are ripe. Visitors may have the opportunity to taste the grapes in the field and perhaps even pick them side by side with the field workers, or take a step-by-step tour of the wine-making process—complete with tasting!

Travel to other countries is not the only way to capture aspects of one's heritage. Tours within the United States are also popular. Many boomers reconnected with distant relatives when they went to Louisiana, Mississippi, and Texas to help during the aftermath of Hurricane Katrina. Trips to Appalachia to learn about the music, dance, or quilting, as well as trips to reservations to learn about the residents' "modern" ways of life or even recapture some of the "old" ways or outlook, are also of interest.

Baby boomers find heritage festivals interesting when they can go in small groups. Travel to events like the Scottish Highland Games, Puerto Rican Days, or a Vietnamese New Year celebration may be attractive to boomers even if they are not of those heritages.

FIELD-TO-PLATE TRAVEL

In an interesting twist on fine dining, a small but fast-growing part of the travel industry is labeled "field-to-plate." This type of event is a response to a desire to reconnect with a simpler life, a rising interest in eating a healthier diet, and zest for a "new" experience. Participants travel to a farm where produce is picked right from the field, prepared on the spot, and served to them on-site—often on tables set up in the field from which the produce has been picked.

This phenomenon is growing in all parts of the United States. A couple of examples come from California and Connecticut. California's Pitchfork and Plate offers many programs, including the following, called "Chef in My Garden!":

> Join some of the most innovative chefs of our region as they create exquisite meals using seasonal, local ingredients paired with the region's best wines, in intimate settings of our region's most interesting garden spaces. (www. plateandpitchfork.com, Home page)

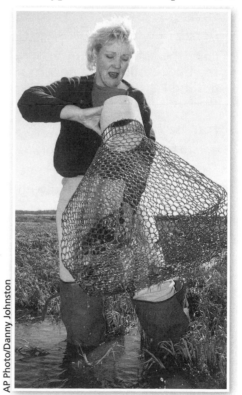

AP Photo/Danny Johnston

Field-to-plate travel presents new and interesting experiences. Nothing says "organic" like catching and preparing your own crawfish!

Also check out Dinners at the Farm, which holds dinners outdoors on 10 different farms over the course of the summer (http://dinnersatthefarm.com), and Outstanding in the Field (www.outstandinginthefield.com). Each uses a slightly different format from Pitchfork and Plate.

In addition to traveling to sites already in operation, check out local possibilities. A caterer may team with a local farmer to provide a similar event near your hometown. A different twist might be to engage the participants in preparing the food themselves.

TRAVEL PROGRAM IDEAS

The following program descriptions will give you some ideas for travel with boomers. Getting ready to go, driving off the beaten path, traveling with grandchildren, and sampling food at the destination site are experiences that boomers crave. Keep in mind that these programs should have an educational component and that the baby boomers like a bit of pampering.

SHUN PIKING: TAKING THE ROAD LESS TRAVELED

> *Description*

Shun the "pike"—get off the main highway and discover the jewels along the back roads. Learn how to prepare for shun piking and how to avoid getting lost. Learn how to read a road map—and fold it back up! Discover the best-kept secrets in the local countryside.

> *Purpose and Goals*

* To become aware of safety precautions when traveling off the main roads
* To learn how to read a map
* To become acquainted with fun and interesting places to visit in the local area

> *Length and Format*

About 1 hour

> *Space*

Quiet room with comfortable seating for all participants

> *Staffing*

One presenter

> *Equipment and Materials*

* Road maps of local area
* Possibly a PowerPoint slide show with pictures of local places to visit (if slides are not shown, an Internet tour can be projected on the screen or a handout can be provided)
* Laptop computer and data projector if PowerPoint is to be used
* Screen

> *Implementation*

    1. Offer a map-reading workshop for those who need tutoring.

    2. Content should include colorful slides of fun out-of-the-way places to visit, to be shown during discussion of the features of these places.

    3. Be sure to address road and travel safety.

    4. Provide a handout of cool places to visit.

> *Options and Variations*

    * Usually a local shun piker can be easily found. These folks enjoy sharing their experiences.

    * An American Automobile Association staff member may be willing to talk about back road safety.

    * Participants can each have in mind two or three places off the beaten path to share with the group.

    * An Internet homework assignment can be completed to check out events happening in small towns in the area (antique fairs and flea markets, little-known historic sites, festivals, scenic drives and views, and so on).

ESCAPE FROM THE EVERYDAY

> *Description*

Take a one-day mini-vacation and escape from the mundane. A variety of workshops will be available—or just relax and enjoy the nature around you.

> *Purpose and Goals*

To have a retreat experience that breaks the daily norm in a drastic way. Focus can be on cuisine, ecology, methods of daily tasks, spirituality, history, special interests, and many other topics. (Survey your participants to become familiar with their interests and incorporate several into one overnight. See "Options and Variations" for activity ideas.)

> *Length and Format*

One to two days

> *Space*

Plan your retreat at a location approximately 1 or 2 hours away. You can host it at a lodge, hotel, or campground; become familiar with the more interesting lodging options in your area. Rooms for workshops will be needed, as well as larger gathering places for the entire group.

> *Staffing*

About one staffperson to 10 participants

> *Equipment and Materials*

Will depend on the types of activities conducted

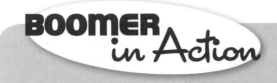

BOOMER in Action

Donna Brannon

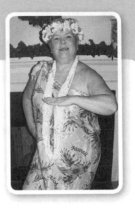

Both friends and family looked at me like I had three heads when I told them I was taking hula dancing lessons. It all started when I joined a line dancing group to get some exercise. The instructor was Hawaiian and asked some of us if we'd like to try hula. I laughed about it and joined only because I really admired my instructor and didn't want to hurt her feelings, but I had no idea it would turn into such a fun and engaging hobby.

At first our group looked like a comedy act, but now our performances have actually become very graceful. Our group's name in Hawaiian means graceful grandmothers.

Who would have ever guessed that I would have danced on stage at Waikiki Beach and at a luau in Maui? The women in our group are like a bunch of little girls—we get so excited about what to wear. We have to get our instructor's approval on our attire because we tend to get carried away with our various costumes, which we make ourselves. She reminds us we must follow Hawaiian tradition.

Hula not only improves coordination (you must use your hands and feet at the same time as well as torso), but it is also a complete exercise for both the mind and body (much like yoga). In hula dancing, hand movements explain words of the songs, much like sign language. When you have truly learned the song, you become most graceful with your movements. You become relaxed and it releases a feeling of well-being. This is why I love hula so much—it doesn't matter if you are overweight (in Hawaii they say they like their women a "healthy size").

Profile and photo courtesy of Donna Brannon.

➤ Implementation

1. Allow participants to provide their own transportation to the retreat, and offer reception hours for their arrival on Friday from 7:00 p.m. to 9:00 p.m. Refreshments or a cocktail hour can facilitate socialization and generate excitement about the weekend.

2. Have an orientation, preview the offerings, and introduce the staff and the planned schedule.

3. An interactive activity should follow.

> *Options and Variations*

Many themes are possible.
>> ***Sample theme:*** Raw food retreat

>> ***Purpose:*** To learn about the benefits of raw food, practice techniques of preparing raw food meals, and experience the benefits of eating a raw food diet for a weekend

>> ***Guest lecturers:*** Local co-op owner to discuss health food benefits and offer fresh fruit and vegetable co-op memberships; raw foods chef (call local vegan or vegetarian restaurants) to prepare meals and teach a cooking class; yoga instructor to lead daily yoga and meditation

GETTING READY TO TRAVEL ABROAD

> *Description*

Traveling to other countries takes planning and preparation. In this session, seasoned travelers will share how to prepare, what to take, what to see, and what to do. How to go through Customs, how to pack, how to exchange money, how to ensure your personal safety, and whether or not to bargain when shopping are just a few of the practicalities you'll explore.

> *Purpose and Goals*

To learn how to prepare for a safe, satisfying adventure in another country

> *Length and Format*

One 3-hour workshop or two 2-hour workshops

> *Space*

Room with space to show travel items (suitcases, clothing, foreign money, and so on) and to show slides

> *Staffing*

One facilitator with guests to share specific topics

> *Equipment and Materials*

* Computer
* Data projector
* Screen
* Travel items such as personal kit, money belt, camera, suitcase, clothing, passport (plus applications), travel-size personal items, documents needed, travel guides, foreign money; resource handouts

> *Implementation*

Divide the program into at least four focus areas:

1. Before you go: Cover paperwork such as passport application, shots, and other records and forms needed; where to get advance information about places to stay and eat, weather, and so on.

2. Pretrip shopping and packing: Cover items to bring, items not to bring, travel-size personal items, handling of prescription medications, carry-on items, walking shoes, how to pack, gear to bring (camera, rain gear vs. umbrella, hats, sewing kit, first aid items, and so on).

3. On the road or in the air: Discuss travel safety—topics like storing your money, sleeping on the plane, food and water along the way, safe use of ATMs, carrying a purse versus wearing a money belt.

4. While you're there: Cover how to find the cool places to visit that most tourists don't know about, must-see places, themed stops (museums, art, cathedrals, natural areas, fountains, architecture).

> *Options and Variations*
  * Travel agents may be willing to facilitate this workshop.
  * International students from local universities may be willing to talk about travel in their countries.
  * Seasoned travelers can share their pictures (ask them to be brief) and share what they've learned through their travels.
  * Many resources are available on the Internet.

FROM GRAPE TO GLASS

> *Description*

See the inner workings of wine making. Watch the grapes being pressed. Learn about fermentation. Smell the wood of the storage barrels. Learn what's in a name (how different types of grapes are used and how different wines are made). Watch the bottling process. Finish with a taste to find your favorite.

> *Purpose and Goals*
  * To learn about the wine-making process from beginning to end
  * To discern types of grapes and find out why some are used and others are not
  * To have a fun taste test

> *Length and Format*

Session 1-1/2 hours long plus travel time

> *Space*

Winery

> *Staffing*

One instructor

> *Equipment and Materials*

On-site, provided by winery

> *Implementation*

Take a bus trip to a local winery. The owner or wine master can conduct the tour.

> *Options and Variations*

Utilize the knowledge of local wine makers. Make sure they are adept at providing lots of information about wine making and are tolerant of being asked many questions.

FINE DINING—YOU BE THE FOOD CRITIC

> *Description*

Try different foods in good restaurants in the region. Learn what the food critics look for. Each week we will try a different restaurant and rate the food. The owners are providing a discount for us.

> *Purpose and Goals*

* To become acquainted with a variety of regional restaurants
* To expand options for future dining
* To learn how food critics assess food, service, and atmosphere

> *Length and Format*

About 1-1/2 hours per week for six to eight weeks plus travel time

> *Space*

Reserved tables for participants—provided by each restaurant

> *Staffing*

One facilitator

> *Equipment and Materials*

Checklist for rating each restaurant

> *Implementation*

1. Participants can meet at the designated restaurant or may carpool.
2. At the beginning of the first week, review how to critique the restaurants.

> *Options and Variations*

* Trips can be offered once or twice a month, year round.
* The local newspaper food critic may be willing to teach participants what she or he looks for in assessing restaurants and meals.
* Weekly or monthly themes may be a fun alternative (Mexican, Indian, Korean; barbeque for Fourth of July; Valentine's Day).

TRAVELING WITH GRANDKIDS

> *Description*

Travel can provide great bonding adventures for grandparents and grandkids. Successful trips require careful advance planning. Learn how to plan and manage the trip, what to do with cranky grandkids or a cranky grandparent (yourself), how to pack, what to do when it rains, how to decide where to go and what to see, and how to save and share memories of the trip after you go back home.

> *Purpose and Goals*

To get guidance on planning all aspects of travel with grandkids

> *Length and Format*

One 3-hour class or two 2-hour classes

> *Space*

Room with space to show travel items (suitcases, clothing, foreign money, and so on) and to show slides

> *Staffing*

* One facilitator with guests to share specific topics
* Seasoned travelers (grandparents and grandkids) can give firsthand tips and hints

> *Equipment and Materials*

* Computer
* Data projector
* Screen
* Travel equipment such as games to play on the road, maps, cameras

> *Implementation*

Have two sessions or two segments within the same session: one for pretrip planning and one for on-the-road planning. Things to consider:

* Pros and cons of taking one grandchild versus two
* Understanding the preferences, interests, developmental needs, and biological needs of a grandchild
* Setting behavioral expectations
* Planning in advance things to see and do
* On-the-road activities
* Planning time apart (or at least noninteractive)
* Food and snacks
* Burning off your grandchild's excess energy when you're dead tired
* Taking pictures, buying mementos, making memories

> *Options and Variations*

* Different classes can be held for traveling by car, by bus or train, by plane.
* Consider the pros and cons of working with a travel agent who plans intergenerational travel.
* Consider the pros and cons of working with intergenerational tour vendors.

TRAVEL TO VOLUNTEER

Another category of programs focuses on traveling for volunteer purposes. Because baby boomers like to work in small, intimate groups, traveling from a community center and working as a group at a wildlife refuge or a historic site may be just the adventure this population is seeking. Trips may take 2 hours to 2 months or longer. Working with a reputable organization whose staff have experience accommodating travel volunteers will save time and energy and will help address liability issues.

Opportunities vary by region, making it impossible to present specific examples that could be offered anywhere. Instead, the following sections describe kinds of programs available within several key agencies. A bit of research on the Internet at these agencies' Web sites will give you further

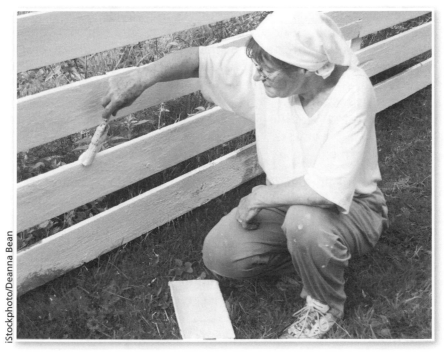

iStockphoto/Deanna Bean

Travel-to-volunteer activities provide many opportunities for folks to meet new people and lend a helping hand.

details and contacts. Keep this in mind: Although baby boomers will work hard, they want to be taken care of. Be sure to feed them well and provide drinks. Make sure that the agency provides proper equipment and instruction for using it safely, as well as supervision.

Travel-to-volunteer opportunities vary greatly. Almost any area of interest is available. Destination sites may give travelers the opportunity to work in health services, for example by assisting with vaccination clinics, eye exams, and well child checks. Construction and reconstruction projects such as Habitat for Humanity are other possibilities, and the projects being completed in the aftermath of Hurricane Katrina still need volunteers. Working with animals such as rescue horses, dogs, cats, and exotic animals is another possibility. Projects related to caring for our natural resources are diverse and are quite popular with baby boomers.

To provide a sampling of travel-to-volunteer projects, the following sections describe programs offered in the natural, historical, and cultural resource areas. Many of these programs are half-day or one-day projects that could be accessed close to home. Others involve stays overnight, over a weekend, or over a longer term. Some agencies provide housing, food, or both. Contact agencies directly for specific information.

Natural Resource–Related Opportunities

Most land use agencies managed by the U.S. government (state and federal) host groups of volunteers. These organizations provide a range of work, involving, for example, guided tours, stocking and staffing "museum" stores, research, land acquisition, resource inventories, special programs, and maintenance. This section highlights a few potential travel-to-volunteer programs for federal land use management, state government, and nonprofit organizations.

The U.S. Fish and Wildlife Service (www.fws.gov) uses volunteers in many capacities. For example, volunteer opportunities in the refuge system include the following:

- Assisting with special events such as Earth Day, various festivals, National Public Lands Day, or fishing derbies
- Conducting fish and wildlife population surveys
- Leading tours and providing information to school groups and other visitors
- Assisting with laboratory research; improving habitat, for example, by reestablishing native plants along a riverbank or eradicating invasive species
- Helping with special projects such as banding ducks
- Performing clerical and administrative duties, for example, staffing an information desk or a natural history "store"

- Working with computers and other technical equipment
- Photographing a variety of natural and cultural resources

Volunteers' skills and interests are generally matched with work opportunities. Many projects require no prior skills.

On-the-job training is provided if needed. For example, volunteers may be trained to identify locally invasive plant or animal species or even endangered species. Locations can be pinpointed via global positioning system (GPS). This information can be entered into a national database that helps the U.S. Fish and Wildlife Service set priorities for eradication of invasive species or protection of species that are endangered.

The following are some specific U.S. Fish and Wildlife Service volunteer projects:

- On the Conte National Wildlife Refuge in Massachusetts each spring, hundreds of volunteers help to stock young Atlantic salmon in rivers and streams throughout the Connecticut River watershed.
- Each year at the Ridgefield and Steigerwald National Wildlife Refuges (Washington State), hundreds of volunteers plant native trees and shrubs at predetermined sites.
- At the Don Edwards San Francisco Bay National Wildlife Refuge (California), volunteers complete projects for habitat restoration including seed germination, propagation of cuttings, transplanting seedlings, pulling weeds, and planting native plants.
- Volunteers at the Aroostook National Wildlife Refuge (Maine) build and place waterfowl nesting cavity boxes, survey to determine mating season use, and resupply clean wood shavings for optimum nesting material.

The U.S. National Park Service holds outstanding resources in trust for the general public. Exemplary natural, historical, archaeological, and cultural resources are preserved, displayed, and interpreted for the public. Multiple volunteer opportunities exist at National Park Service sites across the country. For a complete listing of sites, specific jobs, and contact information, see www.nps.gov/volunteer. The kinds of jobs that groups of volunteers do for the National Park Service include

- conservation education,
- library research,
- visitor information,
- trail and campground maintenance,
- historical preservation,
- construction, and
- weed and other invasive species control.

The following are some specific U.S. National Park Service projects:

- At the Southeast Archeological Center (SEAC, in Florida), volunteers survey and excavate archeological sites under the direction of SEAC archeologists. They can also catalog and curate artifacts and care for the SEAC facility.
- The Point Reyes Morgan Horse Ranch (California) offers volunteers an opportunity to assist in ranch operations. Volunteers care for, handle, and ride horses and clean and maintain tack, equipment, fences, and buildings.
- Volunteers at the Chesapeake & Ohio Canal National Historical Park along the Potomac River (Maryland, West Virginia, and Washington, DC) reendow invasive plant species, paint park structures, work on trail restoration, repair public access trails, remove vegetation from historic structures, paint and repair picnic tables, and install interpretive wayside exhibits.

The U.S. Forest Service also welcomes volunteers interested in natural resource management projects. Opportunities include invasive plant species removal, wetland and pine forest restoration, trail trimming, large-scale trash cleanups, indoor and outdoor painting projects, recycling, and much more. The following are examples of specific projects:

- Visitors maintain trails and do campground maintenance in the Humboldt-Toiyabe National Forest (Spring Mountains National Recreation Area, California).
- Volunteers clear brush and debris from trails, install erosion control devices, and repair bridges in the Willamette National Forest (Oregon).
- In the Gallatin National Forest (Montana), volunteers worked to restore a historic building in the Absaroka-Beartooth Wilderness that had been ransacked by a grizzly bear. In addition to installing new siding and performing cabin maintenance, they built fencing.
- Volunteers and Forest Service archaeologists together survey the areas around Laguna Meadow in the Laguna Mountains (Cleveland National Forest, California). Volunteers and Forest Service staff use handheld GPS to relocate, photograph, and map the sites and note the current conditions of the sites.

Some federal, state, and other agencies work together with volunteers on projects. One such partnership involves the Six Rivers National Forest, Karuk Indigenous Basketweavers, Karuk Tribe of California, California Department of Transportation, and Bureau of Land Management. Volunteers assist traditional basket weavers in collecting, processing, and weaving basketry materials and help prepare for the annual burning of bear grass. A strong educational-cultural component is included, with volunteers also learning about indigenous forest management practices, traditional food preparation, and cultural values.

Additionally, a number of organizations and private nonprofit agencies work with federal agencies to supply volunteers for "working vacations":

- The Sierra Club offers a variety of international and stateside volunteer vacations. Help rehabilitate the forest around the Sierra Club's own Clair Tappaan Lodge in the Tahoe National Forest (California).
- Appalachian Mountain Club volunteers hold regular work parties to help with maintenance and improvement of the trails, shelters, and signs along the Appalachian Trail.
- The American Hiking Club uses the services of small groups of volunteers for trail construction or reconstruction and maintenance or ecological restoration in locations such as the Picketpost Mountain (Arizona), Windham Mountain (Colorado), and Rincon and Tucson Mountain Districts of the Saguaro National Park (Arizona).

State Parks and Forests

Many volunteer opportunities in state parks involve individuals rather than groups and are long-term (e.g., campground host), but many one-day projects also need help. Although opportunities vary by state, common group tasks include the following:

- Trail construction and maintenance
- Native plant enhancement
- Exotic plant removal
- Habitat restoration
- Beach cleanup
- Programs for persons with disabilities
- Historical research
- Restoration of historical structures
- Litter control
- Setting up and monitoring bluebird boxes

These are examples of specific short-term projects:

- At KAMP Dovetail in Ohio's Rocky Fork State Park, volunteers provide summer camp experiences for people with cognitive, sensory, or mobility impairments.
- Regular Volunteer Days are held at the Radnor Lake State Natural Area (Tennessee), where volunteers plant native species, remove exotic plants, and help with other park projects.

- Maryland Department of Natural Resources TREE-MENDOUS program volunteers help restore the natural environment in the Chesapeake Bay area by planting trees.
- Volunteers at the Massachusetts Department of Conservation and Recreation Universal Access program help persons with disabilities and their families and friends enjoy outdoor activities such as boating, fishing, hiking, camping, skiing, and ice skating in the state parks and forests.

Again, the projects listed are just the tip of the iceberg and pertain only to one narrow area of focus. Many other opportunities exist. Check out these Web sites for further details:

www.amcberkshire.org

www.americanhiking.org (click Our Work, then Volunteer Vacations)

www.amizade.org/community_partnerships/montana.html

www.candocanal.org/NPS.html (September 30, 2008)

www.mass.gov/dcr/universal_access/index.htm

www.dnr.state.md.us/forests/treemendous/volunteers.html

www.friendsofaroostooknwr.org/projects.htm

www.fws.gov/desfbay/volunteer.html

www.fws.gov/refuges/profiles/index.cfm?id = 53590

www.lcrep.org/vol_opportunities.htm

www.volunteer.gov/gov/xEventsZ.cfm?myDate = 6/9/2006&month = 6/9/2006&ShowList = Yes

www.nps.gov/seac/

www.passportintime.com/

MARKETING TIPS

The travel industry invests millions each year in marketing and promotions. According to *Ad Age* magazine, most travel businesses spend about 10 percent of their gross revenue on advertising and marketing. Southwest Airlines alone spent almost $175 million on advertising in 2007 (www.adage.com/datacenter, June 23, 2008).

Whether you develop independent travel programs for boomers or create cooperative relationships with travel partners, marketing must be a top priority. For businesses from online travel sites to independent travel agents, the competition is fierce in this growing industry. To succeed as a travel provider for the lucrative baby boomer market, the key is to offer something special, unique, or exclusive.

- **Stay true to your mission:** Your organization has a mission or purpose that should drive all of your programming decisions. Never develop a set of programs or products simply because "everyone else is." In every case, your programs and services must meet the mission of your organization. There are many travel-related businesses in your community and online, but there is no need for you to directly compete with these generic travel providers. Public park and recreation agencies should never compete head-on with private sector travel businesses unless they are filling a community need left unmet by the private sector.

- **Collaborate with travel professionals:** Meet with these professionals to think about ways you can augment and enhance existing trips and tours. Perhaps you can add new value for a cruise group by offering to assist those who have special needs associated with aging. Therapeutic recreation professionals should consider building partnerships with travel agents, tour providers, destination management companies, or hotel concierges. Together you can ensure that boomers, now and in the future, are getting recreational needs met at home and on the road.

- **Position yourself away from travel agents:** You are much more than a travel company. You are an organization dedicated to enhancing quality of life. For many boomers, travel will likely become more than a way to fill leisure time. Rather, travel will be filled with adventure, enrichment, challenges, and self-discovery. When promoting travel-related programs, make sure you are shining the light on the benefits of travel as it relates to health and wellness.

- **Think about specialty travel:** Focus on your expertise when developing a travel program. For example, if your agency is well positioned as a fitness provider and is well staffed with fitness experts, consider developing trips with a fitness focus. Or you may have a thriving adult soccer program, which could inspire a trip to the World Cup. Perhaps you have a following among arts and crafts enthusiasts. Bring them together to plan a trip to a regional or world artistic hub, anywhere from Santa Fe, New Mexico, to Florence, Italy. The key to this type of programming is to include customers in the planning stages so that the trip becomes their trip, rather than yours.

- **Consider medical tourism:** Medical and dental health care consumers are taking their business out of state and out of the country more and more often. As you've learned, baby boomers, wishing to look and stay young forever, will dramatically outspend previous generations on both surgical and nonsurgical cosmetic procedures, ranging from hair transplants to tummy tucks. Often cosmetic procedures are the impetus for a nip–tuck vacation to a luxurious spa. The economy may shift, but vanity will remain. It may also be possible for recreation and leisure agencies to work with cosmetic surgeons in their local area to add a bit of rest and recreation to surgical recovery programs.

- **Market "stay-cations" and "play-cations":** The summer of 2008 saw the emergence of new terms and trends related to vacationing in America. As gas prices pushed past the $4.00 mark for the first time, people were parking their cars, canceling road trips, and rediscovering local treasures. From finding hidden trails and going to concerts in the park to enjoying previously undiscovered eateries and museums, Americans were taking refuge and relaxation in their own neighborhoods and within their own zip codes. People began to consider long-distance travel as an assault on the environment as the notion of global warming crept into conversations from coast to coast.

- **By economic necessity, people realized that eco-travel and adventure travel need not mean planes, trains, or even automobiles.** Look for the travel concept to become less about distance and more about experience. Market the "stay-cation" concept as part of your branding, and you're sure to make an impact on boomers—especially those dealing with shrinking retirement incomes.

10

The Boomer Future

• • • • • • • • • • • • •

So what does the future hold for baby boomers? While no one has a crystal ball, there are many trends driving boomer behavior. Not all of the trends affect boomers alone. Some, like the trends toward mobile media and our obsession with looking good, apply to society at large. But because boomers represent the largest generation alive today, they will continue to move into the spotlight for all types of organizations, both in and out of the leisure and recreation sectors. The following 10 major trends are ones that many foresee as affecting the recreation professional.

① THE BIG BUSINESS OF BOOMERS

Face it! Boomers are the new "cool." But with this realization, you as a park and recreation agency will face an increasing amount of competition for their interest, attention, and participation with each passing day.

As reported in the Financial Times, "By 2015, boomers will have a net worth of some $26 trillion—equivalent to a year's gross domestic product for the U.S. and European region combined. They will control a larger proportion of wealth, income and consumption than any other generation in the country—the first time that consumers over 50 have held such sway over the world's largest economy" (Guerrero & Birchall, 2007).

Boomer conferences seem to be popping up around the world at a frantic pace. One of the first in this category, Boomer Summit brings together journalists, researchers, policy makers, and business professionals to discuss the business of baby boomers.

The American Association of Retired Persons (AARP), a major Boomer Summit sponsor, was joined by others, such as financial services groups, that have long targeted mature adults. Among other major sponsors, however, were media, communications, and technology companies, which in the past have primarily set their sights on young adults and teenagers. Business giants such as Microsoft, Yahoo, and Verizon Wireless are keenly aware of the big business that boomers represent. By sponsoring events targeted to baby boomers, large companies and small can position themselves as boomer friendly, in the same way that others have positioned themselves as family friendly.

While many of the largest for-profit fitness centers are trying to attract older adults, most of their marketing tends to focus on buff "20-somethings." However, with the help of organizations such as the International Council on Active Aging (ICAA), those involved in the public and private fitness industry are gaining new insights into reaching baby boomers and seniors in mutually beneficial ways.

Says ICAA's founder and CEO, Colin Milner (2008), "The concept of 'active aging' goes beyond physical fitness and can be summed up in the phrase 'engaged in life.' No matter their age, people can participate in life as fully as possible, regardless of socioeconomic status or health conditions, within the wellness dimensions." The council's growing membership is composed of businesses, media, agencies, and professionals committed to "changing the way people age by staying active, to the fullest extent possible, within all areas of life: physical, spiritual, emotional, intellectual, professional and social."

The opportunities presented by fitness-seeking baby boomers have led to a growing group of niche gym operators dedicated to serving the 50+ and senior markets. Players include Healthfit, Club 50, and Nifty after Fifty.

According to its Web site, Nifty after Fifty is not just a fitness center for individuals or "baby boomers" who are 50 years and older. It is a full service state-of-the-art fitness center promoting "greater wellness and lasting independence." The Web site also lists a variety of value-added services such as a complete on-site physical therapy service. Nifty after Fifty ultimately brands itself as "much more than a Fitness & Wellness Center. . . . It is a place where you can revive, refresh and take charge for a richer and more rewarding rest of your life" (Zinberg, 2008).

② LIFE IS AN ADVENTURE: ACTIVE RECREATION TOPS BOOMER LIFESTYLE DESIRES

In 2007 an extensive survey of over 5,000 older adults, conducted by the Pro-Matura Group in conjunction with Pulte Homes, Inc., revealed some surprising things about the lifestyle interests of older adults in the United States. The results challenged conventional thinking about "senior recreation." Overall, the survey showed that while interest in many passive recreation activities prevails, adventurous activities such as hiking and river rafting are quickly gaining popularity among the 55-and-over crowd. The survey also confirmed previous findings that health and fitness activities, including strength training and cardio workouts, continue to top the list of leisure interests.

Adventure Activities Emerging

Swimming, golf, and bowling ranked highest among sports, athletic, and outdoor pursuits; but surprisingly, adventure activities like kayaking, hiking, and even hang gliding are quickly working their way up the scale. Hang gliding/parasailing/parachuting was ranked as "extremely important" as a lifestyle offering by 6 percent of the respondents—nearly equal to the 6.1 percent of respondents who ranked competitive running the same.

Team sports like softball and tennis also ranked high. Nearly 20 percent of respondents ranked softball as extremely important, and nearly 25 percent ranked tennis the same.

Leading the charge with adventure programming is Del Webb's Anthem Ranch outside Denver, Colorado, where lifestyle director Scott Hysler has implemented skydiving, white-water rafting, hot air ballooning, sports flying, hang gliding, and even parachuting adventures.

Additionally, according to the national director of lifestyle operations for Pulte Homes, Judy Julison, "The world record for senior rollerblading was set at Sun City Huntley in Huntley, Illinois. I believe we will continue to see activities emerge that reflect this newer interest in adventure and other forms of active versus passive recreation pursuits" (Pulte Homes, 2007, "Press Room"). Table 10.1 reflects the survey responses.

Table 10.1 Top Sports, Athletic, and Outdoor Adventure Pursuits for Those Aged 55 and Older

Activity	Percent ranked "extremely important"
Swimming	55.2
Golf	49.2
Bowling	34.4
Fishing	30.1
Canoeing, kayaking	26.2
Increasing in popularity	
Hiking, climbing, rappelling	18.0
River rafting	17.8
Downhill skiing	9.1
In-line skating	7.3
Competitive running	6.1
Hang gliding, parasailing, parachuting	6.0
Total respondents	**3,584**

Health and Fitness Still Strong

Confirming the importance to this demographic of staying in shape, working out remains a top priority for mature adults. Approximately 77 percent of respondents to the survey indicated that they worked out at least three days per week, and fewer than 6 percent indicated that they worked out zero days per week.

Among health- and fitness-related activities, walking and cardiovascular equipment workouts (e.g., treadmills) top the list. Balance training programs such as Pilates, tai chi, and yoga are on the rise, with more than 51 percent of respondents saying that these were extremely important to programming.

Although active older adults have health and fitness interests aligned with those of past years, there is an emergence of new or broadened programming pursuits and a shift in lifestyle priorities. Lifestyle experts at Pulte Homes' retirement communities have seen a trend of residents still working, therefore, like Del Webb's Bridgewater outside Detroit, Michigan, their fitness facilities get a "workout" earlier in the morning and later in the evening than those communities with a higher percentage of truly "retired" residents. Bridgewater residents tend to use the facilities before and after work, with a general peak in late afternoon and early evening, compared to the traditional model of peak facility use during the 9 a.m. to 5 p.m. workday. Table 10.2 reflects the survey results.

Table 10.2   Top Health and Fitness Pursuits for Those Aged 55 and Over

Activity	Percent ranked "extremely important"
Walking	82.0
Workouts on cardiovascular equipment	78.8
Health and fitness immunizations	68.7
Workouts on strength and weight-training equipment	67.4
Water aerobics exercise classes, water-based fitness	63.0
Swimming	62.5
Increasing in popularity	
Biking	56.7
Balance training programs (yoga, tai chi, Pilates)	51.3
Personal training	41.8
Spinning	18.1
Total respondents	**3,941**

Golf Still Integral to Programming

Golf remains a popular pastime with mature adults. Nearly 40 percent of the survey respondents indicated that they played seasonal golf at least one time per week, and nearly 65 percent indicated that they played at least occasionally. This compares to a 12.3 percent participation rate for people the same ages from the general population of the United States as reported by the National Golf Association. Only 36 percent of those surveyed said that they never played golf (Pulte Homes, 2007).

Men, however, were overwhelmingly more frequent golfers than women. More than 71 percent of men indicated that they played seasonal golf at least occasionally, with nearly 46 percent saying that they played at least one or two times per week. More than 56 percent of women indicated that they played at least occasionally, with 33 percent saying that they played at least once or twice a week. Table 10.3 is reflective of the survey responses.

Table 10.3 Frequency of Playing Golf for Those Aged 55 and Over

Frequency of play	Respondents
Never	35.5%
Less than one time per week	24.6%
One or two times per week	21.1%
Three or four times per week	15.1%
Five or six times per week	3.3%
Seven times per week	0.4%
Total respondents	**3,584**

Crafts and Media Outlets

Although the trend is toward more active recreation opportunities, passive recreation options are still integral to recreation programming. Creative outlets are seeing an increase in demand as well as increasing interest in technology among the demographic.

Besides computer technology, mature adults look for creative outlets such as ceramics, pottery, and claywork; painting and drawing; and wood crafting. The new fad of scrapbooking is on the rise within the group; 16 percent of respondents indicated that it was extremely important. See table 10.4 for the survey responses.

Overall, the ProMatura survey leads to the conclusion that recreation programmers need to encompass multiple dimensions of health and wellness and to respond to new trends and interests that may emerge.

Table 10.4 Top Crafts and Media Outlet Pursuits for Those Aged 55 and Older

Activity	Percent ranked "extremely important"
Ceramics, pottery, claywork	28.4
Painting and drawing	27.2
Wood crafting	27.1
Stained glass making	26.9
Knitting	22.8
Total respondents	**3,204**
Top media and technology pursuits	
Computer technology—general	44.4
Photography	33.5
Computer graphics	33.2
Total respondents	**3,536**

Daniel Rexford (2008), former chief marketing officer of Erickson Retirement Communities, has been conducting research related to the needs of retirees for over 18 years and agrees. "Convergence is key! Organizations that want to be successful with retirees will expand their offerings—diverse disciplines will converge around creating an experience for their clientele. For example, successful fitness organizations are bringing together personal training, physical therapy, nutrition services, yoga, Pilates, instructional and educational programs, clothing, etc."

③ LOOKING GOOD, FEELING OKAY

As with everything else, boomers will reinvent the business of health care. As evident already with the popularity of holistic and alternative therapies, boomers will reach beyond traditional medicine, challenging pharmaceutical, insurance, and medical practitioners to improve everything from customer service to ethics. These new pressures will create opportunities for recreation agencies that are willing to provide programs and position themselves as part of the health care and wellness team.

In 2005, Harris Interactive conducted a study based on online interviews of more than 1,800 Americans between the ages of 41 and 69. According to this research, the greatest fear that baby boomers have, both financially and in terms of lifestyle, involves diminishing health along with health care costs. Further, if knowledge is power, then the Internet has created a new powerful means of access to sophisticated health care information, allowing boomers to take better control of their health futures.

As the human body ages, metabolism slows and systems deteriorate. Of course, study after study shows that healthy, active lifestyles can lessen the negative impacts of the aging process and enhance quality of life. But as boomers begin to reach their 70s and 80s, they will go through many stages of health and wellness. Arthritis and other types of joint diseases affect one's ability to move, exercise, and play. Injuries related to decreasing bone density will heal with the help of all types of medical, physical, emotional, and recreation therapy. Those suffering from major illnesses such as heart disease, stroke, and cancer may seek and benefit from a whole new set of recreation offerings. Even people dealing with emotional conditions associated with aging, such as depression, grief, and anxiety, can turn to recreation and community organizations for support and service.

A report released in 2008 predicted that about 14 million, or roughly 18 percent, of the 76 million baby boomers in the United States can expect to develop Alzheimer's or some other form of dementia in their lifetime. According to the Alzheimer's Association (2008), the direct and indirect costs of Alzheimer's and other dementias to Medicare, Medicaid, and businesses amount to more than $148 billion each year.

Those working in therapeutic and general recreation must prepare for this growing population of people dealing with the emotional and physical effects of Alzheimer's and for their caregivers.

As baby boomers age and face physical health challenges, one thing is clear. They want to look good even if they don't always feel great. In 2006, nearly 11.5 million cosmetic surgical and nonsurgical procedures were performed in the United States, according to the American Society for Aesthetic Plastic Surgery (ASAPS) (www.surgery.org, 2008, "Press"). Since 1997 the overall number of cosmetic procedures has increased 446 percent. The most frequently performed procedure was Botox injections, and the most popular surgical procedure was liposuction. The obsession that baby boomers and their younger counterparts have about prolonging the look of youth has reached epidemic proportions. Recreation professionals will have increasing opportunities to promote active lifestyles and healthy living, not as a replacement for quick cosmetic procedures, but as a way to further enhance body image and reduce the appearance of aging.

The fear of sun-related cancers and other damage becomes increasing prevalent as we age. A common ill effect of outdoor recreation, sun damage can be minimized with the proper precautions. Tennis players, hikers, golfers, and other outdoor enthusiasts will look to recreation professionals and facility designers to help them steer clear of those harmful UV rays. How can you increase the amount of shade and other forms of sun protection to ensure that boomers continue to come outside to play?

④ CONNECTING AND RECONNECTING THROUGH ON- AND OFFLINE SOCIAL NETWORKS

Boomers will spend a good part of their leisure time connecting and reconnecting with friends and family. However, much of the connecting for baby boomers, as well as for younger generations, will take place in virtual worlds and through use of digital media. With applications ranging from social networks to file-sharing sites, from mobile media to smart phone technologies, there is no excuse (whether people would like one or not) for being out of touch. Whether your organization is testing the waters of social networking and mobile marketing or has taken the equivalent of a technological plunge, you must become part of this conversation.

As new communication methods emerge, boomers, although digital immigrants, will eventually embrace these new tools. Never to be outdone by others, baby boomers will come to rely on the same type of instant communication and constant connectivity that their younger, digitally native offspring have always taken for granted.

With reunion sites such as Classmates.com and its rival Reunion.com boasting a combined membership of more than 70 million people in 2008, it's clear that people want to reconnect with friends from their youth. Recreation centers that position themselves as part of this reunion revolution will gain a loyal following among the hippy generation. And romance, both online and off, will be on the radar screen for many baby boomers. Trends

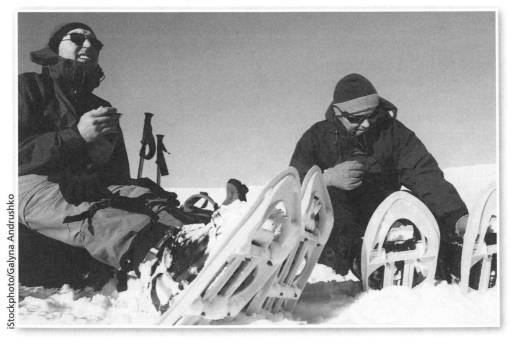

iStockphoto/Galyna Andrushko

Be sure to encourage socializing every step of the way—fun is the name of the game.

related to dating between younger women and older men, Internet dating, and longtime unmarried relationships will also translate into opportunities for recreation centers.

But while the media, Web sites, applications, and technologies are advancing faster than one can type, the fact remains that humans are social beings and like to connect with others in person. Digital connections will never replace a good old-fashioned family or class reunion, and business relationships built online can typically go only so far before parties want to MIRL (meet in real life). Recreation programmers can fill the need for actual connections in real, live spaces.

⑤ TECHNOLOGY TOYS ARE NOT JUST FOR KIDS

According to the Pew Internet and American Life Project (Horrigan, 2008) and 50 + Digital, a consulting firm specializing in media habits of baby boomers, about 70 percent of adults ages 50 to 64 are online; that's 12 percentage points lower than for younger age groups. "However," says 50 + Digital's Mark Miller (2008), "the gap will close as younger Boomers age into the 50 + market. And, as overall Internet audience composition gets more gray, we'll see more use of cutting edge digital applications by 50 + users, including social networking, audio and video and blogs. Companies with the right content and business strategies will find plenty of opportunity to serve 50 + audiences."

Adults are getting tougher to reach through traditional channels such as television, radio, magazines, and newspaper. These are among the findings from the Pew research:

- Adults 25 to 54 spend more time online than do younger demographics—even though the kids are thought of as the Internet generation.
- 42 percent of YouTube's audience is 35 to 54.
- 30 percent of boomers participate in user-generated content, although just 10 percent create content themselves.
- 38 to 40 percent of Internet users are baby boomers.
- Adults ages 35 to 49 are the biggest users of digital video recorders—31 percent use them at least once a week, compared with just 26 percent among 18- to 34-year-olds.

In addition to the amount of time boomers are spending online, they are developing a stronger trust toward online news sources than even television news. During the presidential campaign of 2008, Harris Interactive found that over half of Americans said they tended not to trust the media. More Americans (41 percent) trust Internet news and information sites than trust traditional television news.

With more consumers online and more switching to always-on broadband, the vast majority of marketers will invest a large percentage of marketing moneys in SEO (search engine optimization), banner advertising, and e-mail as part of their media mix.

⑥ WORK IS THE NEW PLAY

In his bestselling book *Microtrends,* Mark Penn (2007) identifies 75 "small forces behind tomorrow's big changes." Penn, like other trend watchers, highlights many trends specific to baby boomers, as well as those affecting society at large. In a section of his book that focuses on trends related to work life, he coins the term "working retired." He says, "Now that so many Americans are living healthily until 85, fewer and fewer actually retire at 65" (p. 29). In 2007 there were twice as many Americans over the age of 65 in the U.S. labor force as in the early 1980s. This shift will have implications not only for boomers, but also for younger generations hoping to move up the corporate ladder and into upper management positions. If older American stay in jobs 10 or even 20 years longer than generations before them, young workers may have fewer, slower advancement options.

But have no fear. It seems as if many boomers may continue to work in a sort of professional volunteer role. Said one young boomer in an online interview, "I love what I do. When I retire I see myself doing the same thing but on my terms and without the pressures of politics and set schedules. I'll be able to do what I love, when I want to do it" (Bonnie, 2008).

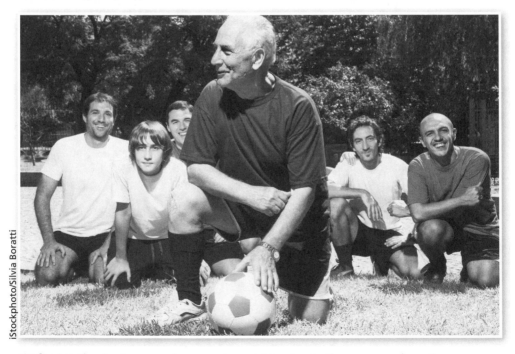

iStockphoto/Silvia Boratti

Professional volunteers, such as coaches, get to stay in the game and continue enjoying a sport they love.

Park and recreation and other community service organizations will greatly benefit from the working retired. However, it will be critical to treat boomer volunteers as valued and esteemed professionals even if they don't get a paycheck or punch a metaphorical clock.

⑦ CAUGHT IN THE MIDDLE: HIGHER EDUCATION, GRANDKIDS, AND CAREGIVING

Caregiving is one of the hottest topics of conversation at boomer social gatherings these days, often surpassing chat about financing university tuitions and downsizing to a condo. According to Mary Furlong (2008), founder of Boomer Business Summit, caregiving is a hot business opportunity as well.

Furlong says that boomers face a new kind of juggling act now that grown children are more independent or on their own. Today a growing number of midlife baby boomers are caring for aging parents or for spouses who are ill or infirm. According to the MetLife Mature Market Institute, 44 percent of Americans over 60 have at least one living parent, up from just 13 percent in 1940. There are 44.3 million family caregivers in the United States who, at an average age of 46, are spending about 34 million hours on the caregiving "job" (Bonnie, 2008). Yet many caregivers still need to keep a day job, save for retirement, run a household, or continue supporting university-age or young adult children. They need help, ranging from respite care to emotional support. Demand is high, and growing, for products and services catering to caregivers' needs, including advice from trusted advisors, in-home support services, help with stress management skills, and long-term care financing.

At the same time, every day in the United States, according to *Grand* magazine, 4,000 moms and dads become grandmas and grandpas at an average age of only 48 years old. Christine Crosby (2008), *Grand*'s founder, says, "Today's grandparents are the hippest, best educated, healthiest and wealthiest generation of grandparents in history." As this demographic explodes, organizations from toy industry marketers to summer camps and cruise companies are starting to realize that their most important revenue growth in the years ahead may come from high-spending boomer grandparents. Especially boomers who may have worked long hours outside the

> **There are only four kinds of people in the world—those who have been caregivers, those who currently are caregivers, those who will be caregivers, and those who will need caregivers.**
> —*Rosalynn Carter, 1997*

home during their own children's formative years may use grandparenting not only to alleviate guilt, but also to connect to their inner child.

Today's boomer grandparents are not only chronologically young but also young at heart. Examples of today's trendy grandparents include Goldie Hawn, Tony Danza, Donny Osmond, Mick Jagger, and Bob Dylan. Today's young grandparents have a lot of time on their hands, shop and research online, and love to spoil their grandkids. This group of superinvolved grandparents opens up new avenues for recreation programmers willing to rethink multigenerational programming and make it more hip, adventurous, and appealing.

When making choices about where, when, and how they spend their leisure time, boomers will demand a new level of convenience and customer service. They will fully embrace Benjamin Franklin's admonition: "Dost thou love life? Then do not squander time, for that is the stuff life is made of." Always a demanding lot, boomers will become even more so as they are pulled in many directions by aging parents, career-seeking children, and almost-perfect grandchildren.

Because boomers will be multitasking on behalf of so many other people, convenience will continue to be a nonnegotiable characteristic of successful products, programs, operations, and services.

⑧ HAPPINESS SEEKERS

Although its pursuit is guaranteed in the Declaration of Independence, happiness is one of the most abstract of all concepts. Baby boomers will pursue happiness in 76 million ways. But, whether the baby boomers you serve are looking to fulfill lifelong dreams, explore new worlds, reconnect with lost loves, or find the true meaning of life, opportunities will abound for parks, recreation, and other boomer-serving organizations.

According to a 2006 study conducted by Leicester University in England, the most significant factors contributing to a country's overall happiness are health, the level of poverty, and access to basic education (Kamenev, 2006). The study also showed that population size plays a role. Smaller countries with greater social cohesion and a stronger sense of national identity tended to score better, while those with the largest populations fared worse. China was #82, India was #125, and Russia was #167 (lower ranking = higher overall happiness). The United States came in at #23, well behind Canada and Costa Rica. Denmark ranked #1. What does a study like this mean to a park and recreation or community services agency? The more you can offer your communities the opportunity to develop community spirit and celebrate the national spirit, the happier they'll be. Though this may be an oversimplification, the study is worth considering especially as it relates to building a loyal, happy boomer following.

As boomers age and physical health deteriorates, self-esteem, confidence, and value will be tested. People will look for happiness through emotional, spiritual, and recreational outlets. Organizations that intentionally make

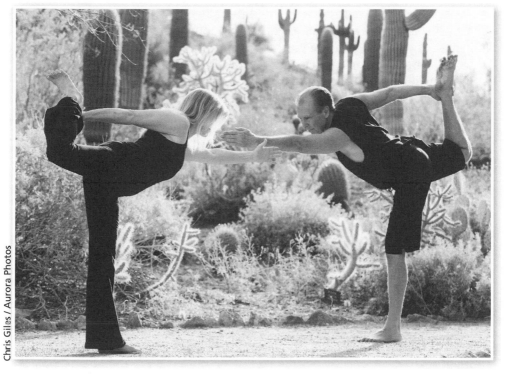

Chris Giles / Aurora Photos

Boomers desire activities that involve the mind, body, and spirit—they want to stay forever young.

people feel good about themselves will thrive. Organizations should focus on making their clientele feel better about themselves rather than on making their clientele feel better about the organization. This is particularly true with retirees. Despite all of their baby boomer bravado, retirees may feel uncomfortable with their perceived loss of influence because they are no longer working. Organizations that are designing programs for baby boomers, especially those who have retired, should think deeply about how they can help customers feel better about themselves.

⑨ LEGACY LEAVERS

Boomers, raised in an era of strong, outward social consciousness that ultimately gave way to a sturdy sense of self, may use their retirement or later years to recapture the selflessness of their youth. Moving forward, "legacy" will be the word of the future as aging boomers grapple with their own mortality, asking questions such as these:

- How can I leave my mark?
- What can I do to make a difference in the world?
- How will I be remembered?

Nonprofits and public agencies will benefit greatly by positioning themselves as legacy makers. Whether you offer boomers a chance to literally leave their mark by offering naming rights to a building, a classroom, a bench, or a tile, or whether you create meaningful opportunities for self-fulfillment, boomers will want to be remembered. You will also want to develop once-in-a-lifetime experiences for boomers looking to have a last hurrah. For example, boomers wishing to fulfill a lifelong dream will pay handsomely to throw out the first pitch at a pro or semipro ball game, play a round of golf with a PGA champion, or play in a band with a classic rock hero.

⑩ NATURAL CONNECTIONS

Since the beginning of time, men, women, and children have longed to connect with nature in meaningful ways. Helen Foster (2008), a longtime specialist in retirement relocation, observes, "It seems that the desire to connect with nature intensifies as we age. So, it's important for residential and community facility developers to make nature easy to see and access."

Foster, who works mostly with mature adults, looks for spaces, buildings, and environments with windows, natural light, courtyards, porches, and balconies. She stresses that walking trails are consistently a top-ranked residential amenity. "The best trails," says Foster, "are not paved paths between buildings, but those which enable a sense of exploration or escape." She adds that the best types of trails also offer view paths, quiet places, and social or activity hubs. Other nature touchstones include natural landscaping, authentically incorporated water features, farm or pasture lands, organic gardening, and other means of connecting to nature. Types of organizations that feed into this quest to connect with Mother Earth include walking clubs and environmental organizations such as the Audubon Society and Sierra Club. Ecological volunteer organizations and farmers' markets also fit into this growing trend.

Mary Lascelles (2008), a relocation specialist in Northern California, agrees with Foster's findings. "I believe that boomers are looking for areas to move where they can enjoy the outdoors as well as theater and good restaurants," she says. In Redding, the area that Lascelles represents, natural attractions involve skiing, snowboarding, fly fishing, hiking, and camping. In addition, Lascelles' clientele cite proximity to cultural centers such as San Francisco, Sacramento, and Ashland in Oregon (popular for its Shakespeare Festival) as critical factors in relocation.

In the Harris study (2005), more than 50 percent of respondents between the ages of 41 and 59 indicated that they would buy a new home for their retirement. Of those, more than 45 percent said that they would move out of state. This number translates to tens of millions of boomers searching for the perfect place to live over the next 20 years. Those communities wishing to attract boomers in the future must invest in recreation services in order to remain viable and competitive.

WHERE DO YOU GO FROM HERE?

While trend information can change before your eyes, there is no denying that aging baby boomers will change your communities and your agencies. The ultimate question, then, is, What will you do with the new ideas and forecasts presented in this book? Will you passively wait for the demands to be met by others? Or will you work now to proactively and diligently develop new programs, products, policies, and conversations to meet this new kind of boomer customer?

As you move forward, it's important to recognize that those around you may not be in tune with this new type of older adult. In order to create change, it may be up to you to educate and inform your community and business leaders about the opportunities and threats posed by the enormous volume of aging boomers. Here are a few ideas to help you begin your boomer recreation revolution:

- Make a commitment to help those around you adapt to this unique population of adults; work with other departments to create a system-wide strategy to meet boomer needs.
- Dedicate a few hours to finding out what resources are available via the Internet that can help you stay on top of future studies and information related to baby boomers.
- Use and share the ideas from this book with leaders, politicians, committees, and staff to help them get on the baby boomer bandwagon.
- Appoint leading-edge and young boomers to existing commissions, committees, and boards that address the needs of "older adults" or "seniors."
- Especially if you are not a baby boomer, get in the habit of reading publications (on- and offline) targeted to baby boomers. AARP is a great place to start.
- Assess your community's resources to learn which organizations are already addressing the needs of baby boomers.
- Begin a conversation with other boomer-minded organizations and individuals in your physical and on-line community to learn how they plan to address baby boomer needs now and throughout the next 5, 10, 20, or even 30 years.

The upside of this boomer focus is that as a recreation organization with an understanding of boomers, you cannot lose! Boomers need what you have to sell and by sheer volume alone can increase everything from program revenue to event attendance and participation. Whether you are one of the 76 million or will spend a majority of your career working with and serving them, boomers will affect the way you live, work, and play. Those willing to become truly boomer centered, adapting to the changing needs of older adults, will be rewarded with loyalty, support, and ultimately success. Get ready for the invasion!

Appendix
Cochran Baby Boomer Quiz*

much has been written about baby boomers; and two elements, the history and societal impact of boomers, became the foundation for the Cochran Baby Boomer Quiz (CBBQ). As a recreation professional with a vested interest in programming, one of the coauthors of this book designed the Cochran Baby Boomer Quiz for two purposes:

1. To evaluate the accuracy of societal norms in relation to baby boomers' knowledge of themselves

2. To evaluate the accuracy of these societal norms in relation to recreation professionals and to measure the professionals' knowledge of baby boomers

Taking into account the unique qualities of the boomer cohort, the Cochran Baby Boomer Quiz is an assessment based on their values of fun and education. Compared to the standard checklist surveys typically used, this provides a means of learning much more about the boomers' values, as well as about what drives their participation in leisure activities.

When we are developing a leisure program, regardless of theory or approach, it is essential to understand the nature of the values within our participants, in this case the boomer cohort. In addition, if values were most important to boomers in their way of life in the past and remain priorities for how they live now, then perhaps recreation professionals should examine these values rather than relying on traditional methods of planning leisure programming or getting lost in the process of deciding what to do with this exclusive cohort. This was the thinking that formed the foundation of this tool.

There are two versions of the Cochran Baby Boomer Quiz, CBBQ-1 (for boomers) and CBBQ-2 (for recreation professionals). The answer key is for the first 26 questions on both versions of the CBBQ.

In both versions, CBBQ-1 and CBBQ-2, the 26 multiple-choice questions were developed from current literature and drew from the four distinct areas of values that make boomers who they are: cultural, social, retirement and leisure pursuits, and economic and educational values.

*Readers are invited to contact the author at lsperazza@brockport.edu with questions about the CBBQ or with results from the quiz to aid in collecting data for continual research.

Table A.1 reflects the linkage of questions to key value words in the literature. It is important to note that although the two tools are similar, each serves a different purpose, allowing for data to be cross-examined; this provides further supportive information for programming with boomers.

Table A.1 Cochran Baby Boomer Quiz: Nonmoral Values as Reflected in the Literature

Value	Question	Key words
Cultural	1	1946-1964
	4	Median age in United States
	8	Boomers over age 50
	17	Ages 65 and older by 2030
Social	2	Age of innocence
	3	Life satisfaction
	12	76 million
	22	Balance, spiritual values
Retirement and leisure	6	Redefine retirement
	9	Individualized activities
	10	Small groups and family
	11	Dedicated to health
	14	Relax, play, and grow
	15	Redefine retirement
	16	Quality, adventure activities
	18	Leisure as necessity
	19	Health club over 55 years of age
	21	Golf in retirement
	23	Retirement destinations
	24	Creating leisure programs
	25	Boomers not with seniors
	26	Involved in sport events
Economic and educational	5	Work, spend, and play hard
	7	Median income level
	13	Education, influential
	20	Spending assets on leisure

In the CBBQ-1 (for boomers), an additional question (part 2, question 1) allows for the collection of extended information on specific leisure values. This question consists of 23 statements (lettered "a" through "w"), each belonging to one of six categories of typical leisure participation nonmoral values (see table A.2). Responses to this question are indicated on a Likert scale ranging from 1 (not important) to 5 (very important).

In both versions of the quiz, the last two open-ended questions (CBBQ-1, part 2, questions 2 and 3; CBBQ-2, part 2, questions 9 and 10) inquire to the activities that boomers *currently* participate in during their leisure time and

Table A.2 Specific Leisure Participation Values

Value	Question	Statement
Competitive	a	To compete against others
	b	Because I am good at it
	c	To show others I can do it
	d	Improve skills or knowledge
	f	For a challenge
	g	For excitement
	w	For risk and adventure
Educational	e	To learn new skills and abilities
	j	To be creative
	v	To expand my intellect
Physiological	k	For physical health or exercise
	o	Relaxation of mind, body, spirit
Social	h	To keep me busy
	i	To help my community
	l	To be with my family
	m	To do things with my friends
	n	To meet new people
	u	For cultural interaction
Relaxation	q	Something different from work
	s	To be alone
	t	To be away from family
Aesthetic	p	Simply for pleasure
	r	To enjoy nature

the leisure activities they *would like to do* during their retirement. The data obtained can be analyzed by categories of leisure activities and frequency for lowest and highest interest levels. Further, these questions were developed to evaluate whether or not current literature is correct (that is, do boomers like to do what the literature says they like to do?).

For recreation professionals, additional questions in CBBQ-2 (part 2, questions 1-8) prompt recreation professionals to rate themselves, their staff, and their agencies on their overall knowledge of boomers and their preparedness for boomers in their facilities, programs, and services. These eight questions were developed based on the author's personal recreation programming experience and other professional experience in the field.

Lastly, both versions of the assessment tool include demographic questions about the respondent's age, gender, and location of residency.

RELIABILITY AND VALIDITY

Both face and content validity were established for the Cochran Baby Boomer Quizzes 1 and 2. Since these quizzes were developed from current published information on baby boomers, they seem to meet the criterion of face validity. Even though face validity is a subjective call and usually is argued to be a weak measure of validity, in the case of Cochran Baby Boomer Quizzes 1 and 2 it is actually a strong reflection of validity because each statement is one that has been written about the boomers.

Additionally, Cochran Baby Boomer Quizzes 1 and 2 show content validity, which was established through a check of the instrument's operation (the content information) against the relevant content domain of the construct, that is, the materials written about the boomers. Content validity is based on the extent to which a measurement reflects the specific intended domain of content and is not a statistical property; rather it is a matter of expert judgment (Vogt, 1999). Again, because Cochran Baby Boomer Quizzes 1 and 2 replicate statements from the literature, content validity is strongly established.

Reliability is the extent to which an experiment, test, or any measuring procedure yields the same result on repeated trials. Both Cochran Baby Boomer Quizzes 1 and 2 call for yes or no answers. With yes or no answers, we must realize that reliability is problematic and is difficult to capture. This does not mean that it cannot be captured, just that a yes or no answer has various implications. Either the subject knew the answer or did not. If reliability is low, we can assume either that subjects did not know the answer or that the question was an unfair question with regard to the knowledge domain. In the case of this study this has great meaning, since we want to learn if what is written about boomers is known by the boomers. Again, since the questions replicate information from a printed source, we assume that they are measuring what is stated in the source.

COCHRAN BABY BOOMER QUIZ I

This baby boomer quiz assesses your current knowledge about the baby boomer generation and your leisure interests. Information obtained from this instrument will aid in the development of programs and services by recreation and park professionals for the baby boom generation.

Directions: Please circle the best answer for each question.

PART I

1. Members of the baby boomer generation were born in which years?
   a. 1935-1952
   b. 1946-1964
   c. 1950-1968
   d. 1960-1976

2. Which "age" is generally associated with the baby boomer generation?
   a. age of innocence
   b. age of rebellion
   c. age of self-indulgence
   d. coming of age

3. Compared with other generations, boomers feel that they have not achieved more and do not have better overall life satisfaction.
   a. true
   b. false

4. The median age of the U.S. population has risen to its highest point in history.
   a. true
   b. false

5. Boomers are known to work hard, play hard, and spend hard.
   a. true
   b. false

6. Boomers lead a busy life and will primarily view retirement as
   a. a transition from society and work
   b. the next stage in their lives to redefine
   c. a midlife crisis

7. The median income level per individual of this age group is
   a. under $50,000
   b. $50,000-$60,000
   c. $70,000-$80,000
   d. over $80,000

From Lynda J. Cochran, Anne M. Rothschadl, and Jodi L. Rudick, 2009, *Leisure Programming for Baby Boomers* (Champaign, IL: Human Kinetics).

8. What percent of boomers were over the age of 50 years in 2005?
   a. less than 20
   b. 35
   c. 42
   d. more than 50

9. Baby boomers enjoy group events rather than individualized activities.
   a. true
   b. false

10. Boomers prefer to socialize in smaller groups and typically stay within extended family circles.
    a. true
    b. false

11. Boomers will remain dedicated to health, wellness, and exercise throughout retirement.
    a. true
    b. false

12. The boomer generation numbers _____ million Americans.
    a. 53
    b. 64
    c. 76
    d. 87

13. Boomers are the most highly educated, influential, and prosperous generation in U.S. history.
    a. true
    b. false

14. Boomers view leisure as only for relaxation or play, not for continued growth.
    a. true
    b. false

15. Boomers will redefine retirement as they have redefined every stage in their lives.
    a. true
    b. false

16. Boomers seek _____ experiences and have the discretionary income to support their desires.
    a. high-quality
    b. adventure
    c. self-fulfilling
    d. all of the above

From Lynda J. Cochran, Anne M. Rothschadl, and Jodi L. Rudick, 2009, *Leisure Programming for Baby Boomers* (Champaign, IL: Human Kinetics).

17. By the year 2030, _____ people will be age 65 years and older.
    a. 1 in 2
    b. 1 in 5
    c. 1 in 8
    d. 1 in 12

18. Though the term *leisure* has a broad theoretical base, it can mean something different to everyone; yet boomers treat leisure as a *necessity.*
    a. true
    b. false

19. Health club memberships for people 55 years and older have _____ over the past 12 years.
    a. decreased
    b. increased
    c. remained steady

20. Boomers will spend the vast majority of their assets on
    a. health care
    b. travel and leisure
    c. investments and income

21. Which of the following is no longer considered the mainstay feature of retirement communities?
    a. fitness centers
    b. walking trails
    c. university courses on-site
    d. golf

22. Boomers are continually searching for balance, lasting relationships, and spiritual values.
    a. true
    b. false

23. Today, what region(s) of the United States is (are) becoming more of a retirement destination than in the past?
    a. Northeast and Southeast
    b. Midwest
    c. Northwest and East
    d. South

From Lynda J. Cochran, Anne M. Rothschadl, and Jodi L. Rudick, 2009, *Leisure Programming for Baby Boomers* (Champaign, IL: Human Kinetics).

24. What factors should be considered when one is programming for the baby boomer generation?
   a. demographic details
   b. attitudes
   c. education and income levels
   d. all of the above

25. Baby boomers should be grouped with seniors in activities despite their legal age and interests.
   a. I agree.
   b. I disagree.

26. Adults ages 35 to 54 are ___ percent more likely than the national average to be involved in some type of sporting event.
   a. less than 6
   b. 12
   c. 25
   d. more than 40

PART 2

1. People have many reasons for participating in leisure activities. How important are each of the following reasons to you? (Please circle one number for each.)

I participate in leisure activities . . .	Not important		Very important		
a. to compete against others	1	2	3	4	5
b. because I am good at it	1	2	3	4	5
c. to show others I can do it	1	2	3	4	5
d. to improve my skills or knowledge	1	2	3	4	5
e. to learn new skills and abilities	1	2	3	4	5
f. for a challenge	1	2	3	4	5
g. for excitement	1	2	3	4	5
h. to keep me busy	1	2	3	4	5
i. to help my community	1	2	3	4	5
j. to be creative	1	2	3	4	5
k. for physical health or exercise	1	2	3	4	5
l. to be with my family	1	2	3	4	5
m. to do things with my friends	1	2	3	4	5
n. to meet new people	1	2	3	4	5
o. for relaxation of mind, body, spirit	1	2	3	4	5
p. simply for pleasure	1	2	3	4	5
q. to do something different from work	1	2	3	4	5
r. to enjoy nature	1	2	3	4	5

From Lynda J. Cochran, Anne M. Rothschadl, and Jodi L. Rudick, 2009, *Leisure Programming for Baby Boomers* (Champaign, IL: Human Kinetics).

I participate in leisure activities . . .	Not important			Very important	
s. to be alone	1	2	3	4	5
t. to be away from my family	1	2	3	4	5
u. for cultural interaction	1	2	3	4	5
v. to expand my intellect	1	2	3	4	5
w. for risk and adventure	1	2	3	4	5
x. other _____	1	2	3	4	5
y. other _____	1	2	3	4	5
z. other _____	1	2	3	4	5

2. What leisure activities do you CURRENTLY participate in during your leisure time?
Please list.

1. _____
2. _____
3. _____
4. _____
5. _____
6. _____

3. What leisure activities WOULD YOU LIKE TO DO during your retirement? These can be the same as those listed for the previous question (just list "same") or can be different.

1. _____
2. _____
3. _____
4. _____
5. _____
6. _____

PART 3

1. What year were you born? _____

2. What is your gender?
   a. male
   b. female

3. What city and state do you currently live in? _____

From Lynda J. Cochran, Anne M. Rothschadl, and Jodi L. Rudick, 2009, *Leisure Programming for Baby Boomers* (Champaign, IL: Human Kinetics).

COCHRAN BABY BOOMER QUIZ 2

This baby boomer quiz assesses your current knowledge about the baby boomer generation and your leisure interests. Information obtained from this instrument will aid in the development of programs and services by recreation and park professionals for the baby boom generation.

Directions: Please circle the best answer for each question.

PART I

1. Members of the baby boomer generation were born in which years?
   a. 1935-1952
   b. 1946-1964
   c. 1950-1968
   d. 1960-1976

2. Which "age" is generally associated with the age of the baby boomer generation?
   a. age of innocence
   b. age of rebellion
   c. age of self-indulgence
   d. coming of age

3. Compared with other generations, boomers feel that they have not achieved more and do not have better overall life satisfaction.
   a. true
   b. false

4. The median age of the U.S. population has risen to its highest point in history.
   a. true
   b. false

5. Boomers are known to work hard, play hard, and spend hard.
   a. true
   b. false

6. Boomers lead a busy life and will primarily view retirement as
   a. a transition from society and work
   b. the next stage in their lives to redefine
   c. a midlife crisis

From Lynda J. Cochran, Anne M. Rothschadl, and Jodi L. Rudick, 2009, *Leisure Programming for Baby Boomers* (Champaign, IL: Human Kinetics).

7. The median income level per individual of this age group is
    a. under $50,000
    b. $50,000-$60,000
    c. $70,000-$80,000
    d. over $80,000

8. What percent of boomers were over the age of 50 years in 2005?
    a. less than 20
    b. 35
    c. 42
    d. more than 50

9. Baby boomers enjoy group events rather than individualized activities.
    a. true
    b. false

10. Boomers prefer to socialize in smaller groups and typically stay within extended family circles.
    a. true
    b. false

11. Boomers will remain dedicated to health, wellness, and exercise throughout retirement.
    a. true
    b. false

12. The boomer generation numbers _____ million Americans.
    a. 53
    b. 64
    c. 76
    d. 87

13. Boomers are the most highly educated, influential, and prosperous generation in U.S. history.
    a. true
    b. false

14. Boomers view leisure as only for relaxation or play, not for continued growth.
    a. true
    b. false

From Lynda J. Cochran, Anne M. Rothschadl, and Jodi L. Rudick, 2009, *Leisure Programming for Baby Boomers* (Champaign, IL: Human Kinetics).

15. Boomers will redefine retirement as they have redefined every stage in their lives.
    a. true
    b. false

16. Boomers seek _____ experiences and have the discretionary income to support their desires.
    a. high-quality
    b. adventure
    c. self-fulfilling
    d. all of the above

17. By the year 2030, _____ people will be age 65 years and older.
    a. 1 in 2
    b. 1 in 5
    c. 1 in 8
    d. 1 in 12

18. Though the term *leisure* has a broad theoretical base, it can mean something different to everyone; yet boomers treat leisure as a *necessity*.
    a. true
    b. false

19. Health club memberships for people 55 years and older have _____ over the past 12 years.
    a. decreased
    b. increased
    c. remained steady

20. Boomers will spend the vast majority of their assets on
    a. health care
    b. travel and leisure
    c. investments and income

21. Which of the following is no longer considered the mainstay feature of retirement communities?
    a. fitness centers
    b. walking trails
    c. university courses on-site
    d. golf

From Lynda J. Cochran, Anne M. Rothschadl, and Jodi L. Rudick, 2009, *Leisure Programming for Baby Boomers* (Champaign, IL: Human Kinetics).

22. Boomers are continually searching for balance, lasting relationships, and spiritual values.
    a. true
    b. false

23. Today, what region(s) of the United States is (are) becoming more of a retirement destination than in the past?
    a. Northeast and Southeast
    b. Midwest
    c. Northwest and East
    d. South

24. What factors should be considered when one is programming for the baby boomer generation?
    a. demographic details
    b. attitudes
    c. education and income levels
    d. all of the above

25. Baby boomers should be grouped with seniors in activities despite their legal age and interests.
    a. true
    b. false

26. Adults ages 35 to 54 are ___ percent more likely than the national average to be involved in some type of sporting event.
    a. less than 6
    b. 12
    c. 25
    d. more than 40

PART 2

1. Has your agency considered the impact that this generation will have on your programs, facilities, and services?
    a. yes
    b. no
    c. somewhat

2. Do you feel that the boomer generation demands more than what our current senior centers and retirement communities are currently providing?
    a. agree
    b. disagree
    c. not sure

From Lynda J. Cochran, Anne M. Rothschadl, and Jodi L. Rudick, 2009, *Leisure Programming for Baby Boomers* (Champaign, IL: Human Kinetics).

3. Do YOU feel confident, with your knowledge about this generation, that you can provide adequate programs, services, and facilities (1 is low, 5 is high)?

      1   2   3   4   5

4. Rate your staff on confidence about this generation and about providing adequate programs, services, and facilities (1 is low, 5 is high)?

      1   2   3   4   5

5. How do you rate your agency's preparedness for the growing aging population and leisure services (1 is low, 5 is high)?

      1   2   3   4   5

6. Several generalizations exist about the baby boomer generation as a whole. Do you feel that adequate research and information are available regarding boomer leisure needs and interests?

    a. Yes, I agree.

    b. No, I disagree—more specific leisure interest research is needed.

7. A program and service guide specific to the baby boomer generation would be helpful to your agency.

    a. agree

    b. disagree

8. What further information do you need from society or the recreation field to adequately meet the leisure demands of the baby boomer generation (for example, income, family, activity interest specifics, demographics)?

9. What leisure activities do you feel boomers CURRENTLY participate in during their leisure time? Please list.

    1. _____

    2. _____

    3. _____

    4. _____

    5. _____

    6. _____

From Lynda J. Cochran, Anne M. Rothschadl, and Jodi L. Rudick, 2009, *Leisure Programming for Baby Boomers* (Champaign, IL: Human Kinetics).

10. What leisure activities do you feel boomers WOULD LIKE TO DO during their retirement? These can be the same as those listed for the previous question (just list "same") or can be different.

1. _____
2. _____
3. _____
4. _____
5. _____
6. _____

PART 3

1. What year were you born? _____

2. What is your gender?
   a. male
   b. female

3. What city and state do you currently live in? _____

From Lynda J. Cochran, Anne M. Rothschadl, and Jodi L. Rudick, 2009, *Leisure Programming for Baby Boomers* (Champaign, IL: Human Kinetics).

COCHRAN BABY BOOMER ANSWER KEY

Responses refer to part 1 of each quiz.

1. Members of the baby boomer generation were born in which years?
   a. 1935-1952
   b. 1946-1964
   c. 1950-1968
   d. 1960-1976

2. Which "age" is generally associated with the age of the baby boomer generation?
   a. age of innocence
   b. age of rebellion
   c. age of self-indulgence
   d. coming of age

3. Compared with other generations, boomers feel that they have not achieved more and do not have better overall life satisfaction.
   a. true
   b. false

4. The median age of the U.S. population has risen to its highest point in history.
   a. true
   b. false

5. Boomers are known to work hard, play hard, and spend hard.
   a. true
   b. false

6. Boomers lead a busy life and will primarily view retirement as
   a. a transition from society and work
   b. the next stage in their lives to redefine
   c. a midlife crisis

7. The median income level per individual of this age group is
   a. Under $50,000
   b. $50,000-$60,000
   c. $70,000-$80,000
   d. over $80,000

From Lynda J. Cochran, Anne M. Rothschadl, and Jodi L. Rudick, 2009, *Leisure Programming for Baby Boomers* (Champaign, IL: Human Kinetics).

8. What percent of boomers were over the age of 50 years in 2005?
   a. less than 20
   b. 35
   c. 42
   d. more than 50

9. Baby boomers enjoy group events rather than individualized activities.
   a. true
   b. false

10. Boomers prefer to socialize in smaller groups and typically stay within extended family circles.
    a. true
    b. false

11. Boomers will remain dedicated to health, wellness, and exercise throughout retirement.
    a. true
    b. false

12. The boomer generation numbers _____ million Americans.
    a. 53
    b. 64
    c. 76
    d. 87

13. Boomers are the most highly educated, influential, and prosperous generation in U.S. history.
    a. true
    b. false

14. Boomers view leisure as only for relaxation or play, not for continued growth.
    a. true
    b. false

15. Boomers will redefine retirement as they have redefined every stage in their lives.
    a. true
    b. false

From Lynda J. Cochran, Anne M. Rothschadl, and Jodi L. Rudick, 2009, *Leisure Programming for Baby Boomers* (Champaign, IL: Human Kinetics).

16. Boomers seek _____ experiences and have the discretionary income to support their desires.
    a. high-quality
    b. adventure
    c. self-fulfilling
    d. all of the above

17. By the year 2030, _____ people will be age 65 years and older.
    a. 1 in 2
    b. 1 in 5
    c. 1 in 8
    d. 1 in 12

18. Though the term *leisure* has a broad theoretical base, it can mean something different to everyone; yet boomers treat leisure as a *necessity.*
    a. true
    b. false

19. Health club memberships for people 55 years and older have _____ over the past 12 years.
    a. decreased
    b. increased
    c. remained steady

20. Boomers will spend the vast majority of their assets on
    a. health care
    b. travel and leisure
    c. investments and income

21. Which of the following is no longer considered the mainstay feature of retirement communities?
    a. fitness centers
    b. walking trails
    c. university courses on-site
    d. golf

22. Boomers are continually searching for balance, lasting relationships, and spiritual values.
    a. true
    b. false

From Lynda J. Cochran, Anne M. Rothschadl, and Jodi L. Rudick, 2009, *Leisure Programming for Baby Boomers* (Champaign, IL: Human Kinetics).

23. Today, what region(s) of the United States is (are) becoming more of a retirement destination than in the past?
    a. Northeast and Southeast
    b. Midwest
    c. Northwest and East
    d. South

24. What factors should be considered when one is programming for the baby boomer generation?
    a. demographic details
    b. attitudes
    c. education and income levels
    d. all of the above

25. Baby boomers should be grouped with seniors in activities despite their legal age and interests.
    a. I agree.
    b. I disagree.

26. Adults ages 35 to 54 are ___ percent more likely than the national average to be involved in some type of sporting event.
    a. less than 6
    b. 12
    c. 25
    d. more than 40

REFERENCES

Active vacations lure fitness minded baby boomers. (2003, March 6). Retrieved October 18, 2004, from www.aarp.org/Articles/a2003-03-06-getaways/tools/printable.

Administration on Aging. (2002). *A profile of older Americans.* Washington, DC: U.S. Department of Health and Human Services.

Alzheimer's Association. (2008). Disease facts and figures. Retrieved March 31, 2008, from www.alz.org/alzheimers_disease_facts_figures.asp.

American Association of Retired Persons. (2004, May). Baby boomers envision retirement II: A survey of baby boomers' expectations for retirement. Retrieved October 18, 2004, from www.aarp.org/research/work/retirement/aresearch-import-865.html.

American Society for Aesthetic Plastic Surgery (ASAPS). (2008). 11.7 million cosmetic procedures in 2007: American Society for Aesthetic Plastic Surgery reports 8% increase in surgical procedures. Retrieved February, 2008 from www.surgery.org/press/news-release .php?id = 491.

Bales, B. (2001, October). Senior fitness. *Parks & Recreation, 36*(10), 96-101.

Bayer, A., & Bonilla, B. (2001, August). Executive summary: Our changing nation. Retrieved October 22, 2004, from www.prcdc.org/summaries/changingnation/changingnation .html.

Belsie, L. (2001, May 15). Boomers reshape culture, again. *Christian Science Monitor, 93*(119), 1.

Bonnie, C. (2008). Media contact. Boomers ready to launch. Retrieved March 14, 2008, from www.metlife.com/FileAssets/MMI/MMICPBoomersReadyLaunchHlghts.pdf.

Borden, N.H. (1964). The concept of the marketing mix. Retrieved February 22, 2008, from www.netmba.com/marketing/mix/.

Carpenter, G., & Parr, M. (2005). Awaken your agency with art: Arts and cultural programming need to have a place in recreation. (Research Update). *Parks & Recreation, 40*(4), 26-33.

CBS News. (2006). The graying of the boomer generation. Retrieved November 3, 2006, from http://cbsnews.com.

Charles, J. (2002). *Moving and being.* Champaign, IL: Stipes.

Cochran, L. (2005). A philosophical and ethical examination of practices in developing leisure program guidelines using the baby boomer cohort. Unpublished doctoral dissertation, University of Idaho, Moscow.

Cochran, L. (2006, October). *What drives boomers to your programs?* National Recreation and Park Association Congress and Exposition.

Crosby, C. (2008). Advertising in Grand magazine. Retrieved March 30, 2008, from www .grandmagazine.com/advertising.asp.

Csikszentmihalyi, M. (1990). *Flow, the psychology of optimal experience.* New York: Harper & Row.

deGrazia, S. (1964). *Of time, work and leisure.* New York: Doubleday.

Demographic profile: American baby boomers. (2003, January). Retrieved August 23, 2004, from www.metlife.com/WPSAssets/19506845461045242298V1FBoomer%20Profile%20 2003.pdf.

Dychtwald, K. (1999). Age power: How the 21st century will be ruled by the new old. New York: Penguin Putnam.

Dychtwald, K. (2005). Retrieved April 8, 2005, from www.aginghipsters.com/blog/archives/000239.php.

Dychtwald, K., & Flower, J. (1992). New leisure. In M.T. Allison (Ed.), *Play, leisure and quality of life* (pp. 349-366). Dubuque, IA: Kendall/Hunt.

Dylan, B. (1964). The times they are a-changin'. Retrieved February 22, 2008, from www.bobdylan.com/moderntimes/lyrics/main.html.

Edginton, C.R., Hudson, S. D., Dieser, R.B., & Edginton, S.R. (2004). *Leisure programming: A service-centered and benefits approach*. (4th ed). New York: McGraw Hill Publications.

Elias, J. L., & Merriam, S. B. (1995). *Philosophical foundations of adult education*. 2nd Ed. Malabar, FL: Krieger.

Elias, M. (2001, February 27). Baby boomers rewrite the rules. Retrieved August 23, 2004, from wwwusatoday.com/life/2001-02-28-baby-boomers.htm.

Fetto, J. (2000, February). The wild ones. *American Demographics, 22*(2), 72.

FH Boom. (2006, November). Survey of U.S. boomers (adults 42-60 years of age). www.theboomerblog.com.

Foster, H. (2008, March 27). Personal communication. Principal, Foster Strategy, New Orleans, Louisiana.

Freedman, M. (1999). *Prime time: How baby boomers will revolutionize retirement and transform America*. New York: Public Affairs.

Furlong, M. (2008). Boomer Business Summit. Retrieved March 30, 2008, from http://boomersummit.com/.

Gaines-Ross, L. (2007). B2F connections. Retrieved March 19, 2007, from http://webershandwick.com.

Gillon, S. (2004). *Boomer nation: The largest and richest generation ever and how it changed America*. New York: Free Press.

Gilmartin, J. (2007). Retrieved February 21, 2008, from www.comingofage.com.

Gilmartin, J. (2008). Retrieved February 1, 2008, from www.comingofage.com.

Godbey, G. C. (2003). *Leisure in your life: An exploration* (6th ed.). State College, PA: Venture.

Guerrero, F., & Birchall, J. (2007, December 5). Boom time. *Financial Times*. Retrieved March 26, 2008, from http://boomersummit.com.

Harris Interactive. (2005, May). Pulte Homes baby boomer study. Retrieved March 18, 2008, from www.pultehomes.com/media.

Harris Interactive. (2008). Retrieved March 31, 2008, from www.businesswire.com.

Herzberg, F., Mausner, B., & Snyderman, B. (1959). *The motivation to work*. New York: Wiley.

Hilton, T. (2005). Personal communication. Howard County, Maryland.

Horrigan, J. (2008). Technology and media use—mobile access to data and information. Pew Internet and American Life Project. Retrieved March 5, 2008, from www.pewinternet.org/.

Iso-Ahola, S. E. (1980). *The psychology of leisure and recreation*. Dubuque, IA: Wm. C. Brown.

Iso-Ahola, S. E., & Mannell, R. C. (1985). Social psychological constraints on leisure. In M.G. Wade (Ed.). *Constraints on Leisure* (pp. 111-151). Springfield, IL: Charles C. Thomas.

Kamenev, M. (2006, October 11). Rating countries for the happiness factor. *BusinessWeek*. Retrieved February 10, 2008, from www.businessweek.com.

Keating, P. (2004, September/October). Wake-up call. *AARP: The Magazine, 47*(5B), 55-60.

Kleiber, D. (1985). Motivational reorientation in adulthood and the resource of leisure. In D. Kleiber & M. Maehr (Eds.). *Motivation and adulthood.* Greenwich, CT: JAI.

Kretchmar, R. S. (2000). Moving and being moved: Implications for practice. *Quest, 52*(3), 260-272.

Kretchmar, R. S. (2004). *Practical philosophy of sport* (2nd ed.). Champaign, IL: Human Kinetics.

Lascelles, M. (2008, March 25). Personal communication. Relocation director/business development, Concierge Relocation Services, Redding, California.

Leading edge baby boomers have specific ideas about retirement. (2001, February). Retrieved October 26, 2004, from www.retirementliving.com/RLart99.htm.

Maslow, A.H. (1954). *Motivation and personality.* New York: Harper & Row.

McGonigal, K. (2007). Facilitating fellowship: Fitness professionals play a key role in helping students and clients reap the many benefits of social connection. *IDEA Fitness Journal, 4*(6), 72-79.

Meisler, J.G. (2003). Toward optimal health: The experts discuss fitness among baby boomers. *Journal of Women's Health, 12*(3), 219-225.

Miller, M. (2008). 50 + Digital. Retrieved March 18, 2008, from www.50plusdigital.com/blog/category/media/.

Milner, C. (2008). Active aging philosophy. Retrieved April 2, 2008, from www.icaa.cc/About_us/ at www.icaa.cc.

Miringoff, M.L., & Opdycke, S. (2005). *Arts, culture, and the social health of the nation 2005.* Poughkeepsie, NY: Institute for Innovation in Social Policy, Vassar College. http://iisp.vassar.edu/artsculture.pdf.

Most, B. (1996, August). Focus: The changing dynamics of retirement. Retrieved October 22, 2004, from www.fpanet.org/journal/articles/1996_Issues/jfp0896.cfm.

National Endowment for the Arts. (2005). Research note #89: Arts and leisure activities: Evidence from the 2002 survey of public participation in the arts. Washington, DC: National Endowment for the Arts.

Neulinger, J. (1974). *The psychology of leisure: Research approaches to the study of leisure.* Springfield, IL: Charles C. Thomas.

O'Keefe, E. (2007). Attention is first. Retrieved January 22, 2008, from www.myprofessionaladvertising.com.

O'Sullivan, E. (2004, October). Action agenda 2000: Trends into practice. Presented at the National Recreation and Park Association Congress, Reno, Nevada.

Parkel, J. (2003, Aug/Sept). The changing face of aging. *Executive Speeches, 18*(1), 28.

Penn, M.J. (2007). *Microtrends.* New York: Twelve Hatchette.

Pieper, J. (1965). *Leisure: The basis of culture.* London: Fontana.

Pulte Homes, Inc. (2007, April 4). Active recreation tops lifestyle desires for over-55 crowd and baby boomers. Retrieved from www.pulte.com at http://phx.corporate-ir.net/phoenix.zhtml?c = 147717&p = irol-newsarticle_print&ID = 981725.

Reunion.com. Home page. http://affiliates.reunion.com.

Rexford, D. (2008, March 28). Personal communication. Former chief marketing officer, Erickson Retirement Communities.

Rossman, J.R., & Schlatter, B.E. (2003). *Recreation programming: Designing leisure experiences.* (4th ed.). Champaign, IL: Sagamore.

Rudestam, K. E., & Newton, R. R. (2001). *Surviving your dissertation: A comprehensive guide to content and process.* (2nd ed.). Thousand Oaks, CA: Sage Publications.

Rudick, J. (2000). *BAM! Benefits activated marketing.* Oceanside, CA: Advisors Marketing Group.

Rudick, J. (2007). *101 marketing essentials every camp needs to know.* Monterey, CA: Healthy Learning.

Thornhill, M., & Martin, J. (2007). *Boomer consumer: Ten new rules for marketing to America's largest, wealthiest and most influential group.* Great Falls, VA: LINX Corp.

Todd, C. (2004, October). Perception is reality. Presented at the National Recreation and Park Association Congress, Reno, Nevada.

Toffler, A. (1990). *Powershift: Knowledge, wealth and violence at the edge of the 21st century.* New York: Bantam Books.

Trump, D. (1989). *The art of the deal.* New York: Warner Books.

Updegrave, W. (2004, August). Ready or not. *Money, 33*(8), 45-49.

U.S. Bureau of the Census. (2000). Retrieved October 15, 2007 from www.census.gov/.

Vogt, W.P. (1999). *Dictionary of statistics and methodology: A nontechnical guide for the social sciences.* 2nd ed. Thousand Oaks, CA: Sage.

Weiss, B. (2005). Personal communication. Recreation director, City of San Carlos, California.

Wolfe, D.B., & Snyder, R. (2003). *Ageless marketing.* Chicago: Dearborn.

World Factbook, The (online). Retrieved October 22, 2004, from www.cia.gov/library/publications/the-world-factbook.

Ziegler, J. (2002, October). Recreating retirement: How will baby boomers reshape leisure in their 60s? *Parks and Recreation, 37*(10), 56-61.

Ziegler, J., & O'Sullivan, E. (2004, October). Serving senior adults—all of them! Presented at the National Recreation and Park Association Congress, Reno, Nevada.

Zinberg, S. (2008). About us. Retrieved March 14, 2008, from www.niftyafterfifty.com.

INDEX

Note: The letters *f* and *t* after page numbers indicate figures or tables, respectively.

ABOUT THE AUTHORS

Lynda J. Cochran, PhD, CPRP, is an assistant professor of recreation and leisure studies at the State University of New York, College at Brockport. A certified park and recreation professional, Cochran has over 10 years of practical experience as a recreation programmer and manager in both municipal and military settings.

As a researcher, Cochran has focused on the study of the leisure values of the baby boomer cohort and applied philosophy in leisure programming methods. She has made several presentations at the local, state, and national levels on programming for baby boomers.

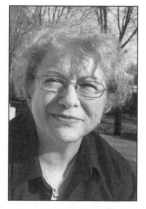

Lynda J. Cochran

Cochran is a member of the National Recreation and Park Association; New York State Recreation and Park Association; American Alliance for Health, Physical Education, Recreation and Dance; and the International Council of Active Aging. She is an active Kiwanis member. In 2002, Cochran received the Meritorious Civilian Service Award, one of the highest civilian honors awarded by the Department of the United States Navy.

In her free time, Cochran enjoys traveling and the outdoor pursuits of golf, swimming, biking, hiking, camping, and geocaching. She and her husband, Thomas Sperazza, reside in Buffalo, New York.

Anne M. Rothschadl, PhD, is an associate professor of sport management and recreation at Springfield College in Springfield, Masssachusetts. Rothschadl has been researching trends and issues of the baby boomer generation for more than 10 years.

Rothschadl has served on the board of directors of the Leisure and Aging section of the National Recreation and Park Association. She has spoken on trends in leisure programming for baby boomers at state and national conferences, including National Recreation and Park Association, National Council on Aging, American Society on Aging, and Canadian Therapeutic Recreation Association. She is also a

Anne M. Rothschadl

facilitator of retirement preparation workshops for Myera, a company that provides planning services for those who are approaching retirement or have recently retired.

In her free time, Rothschadl enjoys traveling, cross country skiing, and Cape Breton-style Scottish fiddling. She resides in South Hadley, Massachusetts.

Jodi L. Rudick, MAS, is president of ADvisors Marketing Group in Oceanside, California. Rudick is a leading marketing consultant, working with everyone from nonprofit organizations to Fortune 500 companies. She is dedicated to promoting participation, advocacy, and support for park and recreation organizations. In 1995, she created the Parks and Recreation: The Benefits Are Endless campaign for the National Recreation and Park Association.

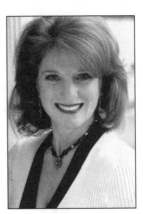

Jodi L. Rudick

Rudick has spoken at more than 250 recreation-related conferences and workshops, including National Recreation and Park Association, and was twice named Speaker of the Year by the Promotional Products Association.

Rudick served on the Oceanside Park and Recreation Commission for six years and currently serves on the City of Carlsbad's Sister Cities Committee. Rudick has also served on the boards of Boys and Girls Clubs, Big Brothers/ Big Sisters, and Meeting Planners International.

In her free time, Rudick likes to watch movies and spend time with her son. She resides in Carlsbad, California.